Changing Social Attitudes Toward Disability

Whilst leg...n may hav...progressed internationally and nationally for disabled people, bar...ontinue to ...xist, of which one of the most pervasive and ingrained is attitudir...ial attitudes are often rooted in a lack of knowledge and are perpetuate...;h erroneous stereotypes, and ultimately these legal and policy changes a...'ual without a corresponding attitudinal change.

This un...rovides a much needed, multifaceted exploration of changing social att...:d disability. Adopting a tripartite approach to examining disability...ooks at historical, cultural, and education studies, broadly conceive...rovide a multidisciplinary and interdisciplinary approach to the docun...endorsement of changing social attitudes toward disability. Written by...of established and emerging scholars in the field, the book aims to br...:me of the unhelpful boundaries between disciplines so that disability is...is...l as an issue for all of us across all aspects of society, and to encourage r...o r.cognise disability in all its forms and within all its contexts.

This truly...idimensional approach to changing social attitudes will be important r...for students and researchers of disability from education, cultural, anc...ility studies, and all those interested in the questions and issues surrounding...les toward disability.

David Bolt is director of the Centre for Culture & Disability Studies, Liverpool Hope University, UK. He is a co-editor of the book series Literary Disability Studies, founder of the International Network of Literary & Cultural Disability Scholars and Editor-in-Chief of the *Journal of Literary & Cultural Disability Studies*. He is also co-editor of the book *The Madwoman and the Blindman* (The Ohio State University Press) and author of *The Metanarrative of Blindness* (University of Michigan Press). Dr Bolt is an editorial board member of both *Disability & Society* and the *Journal of Visual Impairment & Blindness*.

Routledge Advances in Disability Studies

New titles

Towards a Contextual Psychology of Disablism
Brian Watermeyer

Disability, Hate Crime and Violence
Edited by Alan Roulstone and Hannah Mason-Bish

Branding and Designing Disability
Reconceptualising Disability Studies
Elizabeth DePoy and Stephen Gilson

Crises, Conflict and Disability
Ensuring Equality
Edited by David Mitchell and Valerie Karr

Disability, Spaces and Places of Policy Exclusion
Edited by Karen Soldatic, Hannah Morgan and Alan Roulstone

Changing Social Attitudes Toward Disability
Perspectives from historical, cultural, and educational studies
Edited by David Bolt

Forthcoming titles

Intellectual Disability and Social Theory
Philosophical Debates on Being Human
Chrissie Rogers

Disabled Childhoods
Monitoring Differences and Emerging Identities
Janice McLaughlin, Emma Clavering and Edmund Coleman-Fountain

Changing Social Attitudes Toward Disability

Perspectives from historical, cultural, and educational studies

Edited by David Bolt

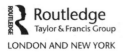
Routledge
Taylor & Francis Group

LONDON AND NEW YORK

First published 2014
by Routledge
2 Park Square, Milton Park, Abingdon, Oxfordshire OX14 4RN

and by Routledge
711 Third Avenue, New York, NY 10017

First issued in paperback 2016

Routledge is an imprint of the Taylor & Francis Group, an informa business

British Library Cataloguing in Publication Data
A catalogue record for this book is available from the British Library

Library of Congress Cataloging in Publication Data
Bolt, David, 1966-
Changing social attitudes toward disability : perspectives from historical, cultural, and educational studies / edited by David Bolt.
pages cm. -- (Routledge advances in disability studies)
1. People with disabilities--Public opinion. 2. People with disabilities in mass media. 3. Sociology of disability. I. Title.
HV1568.B66 2014
305.9'08--dc23
2014000460

ISBN 13: 978-1-138-21605-1 (pbk)
ISBN 13: 978-0-415-73249-9 (hbk)

Typeset in Times
by Saxon Graphics Ltd, Derby

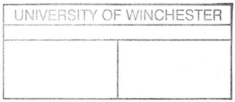

Contents

Acknowledgements   viii

Introduction   1
DAVID BOLT

PART I
Disability, attitudes, and history   13

1 **Evolution and human uniqueness: prehistory, disability,
   and the unexpected anthropology of Charles Darwin**   15
   DAVID DOAT

2 **Killer consumptive in the Wild West: the posthumous
   decline of Doc Holliday**   26
   ALEX TANKARD

3 **'Beings in another galaxy': historians, the Nazi 'euthanasia'
   programme, and the question of opposition**   38
   EMMELINE BURDETT

4 **Disability and photojournalism in the age of the image**   50
   ALICE HALL

5 **Mental disability and rhetoricity retold: the memoir on drugs**   60
   CATHERINE PRENDERGAST

PART II
Disability, attitudes, and culture   69

6   **The 'hunchback': across cultures and time**   71
    TOM COOGAN

7   **Altered men: war, body trauma, and the origins of the**
    cyborg soldier in American science fiction   80
    SUE SMITH

8   **The cultural work of disability and illness memoirs:**
    schizophrenia as collaborative life narrative   89
    STELLA BOLAKI

9   **Impaired or empowered? Mapping disability onto**
    European literature   99
    PAULINE EYRE

10   **The supremacy of sight: aesthetics, representations,**
    and attitudes   109
    DAVID BOLT

PART III
Disability, attitudes, and education   119

11   **Ethnic cleansing? Disability and the colonisation of**
    the intranet   121
    ALAN HODKINSON

12   **Creative subjects? Critically documenting art education**
    and disability   132
    CLAIRE PENKETH

13   **Dysrationalia: an institutional learning disability?**   142
    OWEN BARDEN

14   **'Lexism' and the temporal problem of defining 'dyslexia'**   153
    CRAIG COLLINSON

15 **Behaviour, emotion, and social attitudes: the education of 'challenging' pupils**   162
MARIE CASLIN

Epilogue: attitudes and actions   172
DAVID BOLT

Contributors   176
Index   178

Acknowledgements

I first had the idea for a culturally focused disability studies centre when I was Honorary Research Fellow at the Centre for Disability Research at the University of Lancaster. The idea grew from correspondence with editorial board members of the *Journal of Literary and Cultural Disability Studies* (JLCDS) and conversations with Clare Barker, Lucy Burke, Lennard Davis, Dan Goodley, Petra Kuppers, Rebecca Mallet, Robert McRuer, Claire Molloy, Stuart Murray, Irene Rose, and Carol Thomas.

Thanks to the support and guidance of Ria Cheyne, Peter Clough, Tom Coogan, Heather Cunningham, Ann-Marie Jones, Shirley Potts, and Laura Waite, as well as Tony Edwards, Bart McGettrick, Kenneth Newport, Gerald Pillay, and June Wilson, the idea was put into practice soon after I started working at Liverpool Hope University and founded the Centre for Culture and Disability Studies (CCDS).

As Director of the CCDS I have organised and chaired a series of seminars on which this book is based. I am therefore indebted to everyone who has attended and endorsed the series, from my introductory seminar to the first special guest session with Liz Crow, from the work on attitudes to the current work on voice. I am grateful, too, to James Watson for recognising this work and encouraging me to submit a book proposal to his excellent series.

Half a decade on from starting in my current post, I have also come to rely on my newer Liverpool Hope University colleagues Owen Barden, Marie Caslin, Jessica Chong, Alan Hodkinson, and Claire Penketh – as well as my support worker Philippa Leddra and other supportive colleagues such as Karen Doyle, Siobhan Garber, Marc Jones, Eileen Kavanagh, Chris Lowry, Jacqueline Lloyd, and Christine Parry.

As editor of the book I must thank everyone from whom I have received advice, example, and encouragement on how to go about such work. Tammy Berberi, James Berger, Brenda Jo Brueggemann, Johnson Cheu, Simone Chess, Helen Deutsch, Jim Ferris, Anne Finger, Maria Frawley, Chris Gabbard, Martin Halliwell, Diane Price Herndl, Martha Stoddard Holmes, Richard Ingram, Alison Kafer, Deborah Kent, Georgina Kleege, Fiona Kumari Campbell, Miriamne Ara Krummel, Stephen Kuusisto, Madonne Miner, David Mitchell, Mark Mossman, Felicity Nussbaum, James Overboe, Ato Quayson, Carrie Sandahl, Susan Schweik, David Serlin, Sharon Snyder, Anne Waldschmidt, and the rest of the *JLCDS* editorial board must all be thanked for their general help.

I have also learned much about editing from everyone involved in the *Literary Disability Studies* book series, especially my co-editors, Elizabeth Donaldson and Julia Miele Rodas, and the editorial board members, Michael Bérubé, G. Thomas Couser, Michael Davidson, Rosemarie Garland-Thomson, Cynthia Lewiecki-Wilson, and Tobin Siebers.

Many of these colleagues have become friends and I am lucky, too, to have somehow sustained friendships since childhood. Peter Bagnall and David Cuddy continue to tolerate my fleeting visits to Newcastle Under Lyme, but never fail to please me with their lager-fuelled, joyous company.

All my family should be thanked, but especially my mum, dad, brother Stephen, sister-in-law Gerry, and above all, my daughter Nisha.

Finally, in everything I do I am thankful for the love of my partner, Heidi.

Introduction

Perspectives from historical, cultural, and educational studies

David Bolt

Often contrasted with actions, attitudes are sometimes in danger of being underestimated, deemed relatively harmless. Actions speak louder than words, or so the saying goes, and attitudes tend to be aligned with words more than with actions. But the fact is that attitudes and actions – not to mention words – are intrinsically connected. Problematic social attitudes toward disability, therefore, must be challenged and changed before related actions can become meaningful. For example, in the United Kingdom, those of us who use guide dogs for mobility are well aware that there is now legislation against restaurateurs who refuse our custom, but this does not mark the end of us being made to feel unwelcome in restaurants that are owned or managed by people who have disabling attitudes. Unfortunately, comparable scenarios may be put forward by those of us who have diagnostic labels that pertain to sensory, cognitive, physical, mental, learning, and/or mobility impairments, and may relate to education, leisure, accommodation, employment, and so on. These recurrent scenarios are underpinned by attitudinal barriers and epitomise the anomalous practice to which I return later. The fact is that, although things are slowly changing (Shakespeare, 2006), for centuries, people have been subjected to disabling attitudes, resulting in discrimination and other prejudiced actions, the endeavour to address which has involved the employment of strategies that pertain not only to policy and legislation, but also to language, culture, and education (Isaac et al., 2010; Harpur, 2012). All of these things are explored in this introductory chapter, which provides a brief literature review of work on social attitudes toward disability from the past few decades and culminates in an overview of the book.

Researching disability

Since the early days of disability studies, some of the most eminent figures in the field have problematised the very nature of disability research. The primary concern was that prevalent attitudes toward disability may well have been uncovered as a result of research or social analysis, but those who carried out such work thereby participated in the disabling social relationship (Finkelstein, 1980). Most obviously, researchers who adopted a deficiency perspective were likely to render disability as individual limitations or incompetence (Harrison, 1995). In these terms, knowledge about social attitudes toward disability could not be separated from the conditions in which it was gathered (Finkelstein, 1980). Any such research, moreover, was said to have little influence on policy and to make no contribution to improving the lives of people who were disabled (Oliver, 1992). Disability research was deemed at best irrelevant and at worst part of the social problem, contributing, as it did, to an environment increasingly identified as disabling.

Thankfully, some of these issues were addressed by methodological diversity. Before the 1990s, usually based on quantitative empirical studies, researchers who took various theoretical approaches assumed that attitudes toward disability were pejorative and prejudiced. This was the premise of a review that argued that much attitudinal research was based on a simplified if not simplistic notion of both attitudes and methodology (Söder, 1990). These limitations notwithstanding, an interpretation was posited that moved away from prejudice and toward ambivalence, whereby attitudes were explained as a result of conflicting values that were widely shared in culture (Söder, 1990). The aim was to problematise the supposed stability and individuality of attitudes and trace the link with societal ideologies. Moreover, although a tradition in social psychology had been to use rating scales, it was subsequently suggested that qualitative research methodology would give a richer, more rounded account of attitudes toward disability (Deal, 2003). These studies resonated with the British social model of disability insofar as they helped to recognise environmental rather than individual locations of disabling attitudes. Indeed, the growing appreciation of the radical social model in the 1990s had a significant impact on researchers who, rather than following the interests of politicians, policy makers, and professional academics, began to pursue an emancipatory disability research agenda (Barnes, 2003). Contrary to the primary concern about disability research, the contention was that, when directly linked to the on-going struggle for change, emancipatory work would influence policy and thus contribute to improving the lives of people who were disabled.

Though variously addressed in the past few decades, the problematics of disability research have not yet been eliminated. In the United Kingdom, due to a lack of robust evidence and effective survey research methodologies, the agenda of social justice for people who are disabled remains far from satisfactory (Purdam et al., 2008). In the United States, there is a growing use of what we may think of as concerning methodologies – namely, participatory research, client-based research, community consultation, and so on (Snyder and Mitchell, 2006). Reminiscent of the primary concerns about disability research, the worry about these methodologies is that we risk reproducing something of the very structure that disability studies is meant to challenge. The present book, therefore, accords with the contention that textual analysis provides a remedy to the exhaustion of people-based research (Snyder and Mitchell, 2006). The rationale is that, exhausting only the researcher, this kind of work provides close and revealing readings of cultural texts that are products of the society that has been recognised as disabling. That is to say, representational methodologies offer a way of exploring social attitudes toward disability without contributing to the ableism and disablism at their very core.

Ableism and disablism

As a result of research on disability in the United Kingdom, it has been suggested that the development of a common language with which people who are disabled and people who are not disabled can discuss issues around impairment, disability, and exclusion is a prerequisite for any practical work on changing attitudes (Tregaskis, 2000). In this vein I must refer us to two important terms that are used in the present book. First, defined as a political term used by people who are disabled to call attention to assumptions about normalcy (Davis, 1995), *ableism* is adopted by a number of academics in the west (Campbell, 2008; Bolt et al., 2012; Harpur, 2012). Second, on a par with *sexism, racism,* and *homophobia* (Thomas, 2004), *disablism* is used by some people to denote issues of exclusion (Deal, 2007; Madriaga, 2007). These critical concepts may be thought of as two sides of the same ideological coin: ableism renders people who are not disabled as supreme; disablism refers to attitudes and actions against people who are disabled. In other words, ableism is to disablism what patriarchy is to misogyny.

Here, we can barely begin to explore the many and varied ways in which ableism and disablism are institutionalised. Most obviously, language is a fundamental aspect of the culture by which society is defined. So if we analyse terminology, we learn much about changing social attitudes. For example, the journal we now all know as *Disability and Society* was first published, in 1986, under the title *Disability, Handicap and Society*. The titular modification was made in 1993 and as such was indicative of attitudinal change that had been documented within the first decade of production. An empirical study found that the term *learning difficulties* was associated with more positive attitudes than *mentally handicapped*; that there were no significant differences between the terms *mentally handicapped* and *mentally subnormal*; and that discovering that new neighbours had learning difficulties would have led to a greater level of acceptance than if they were termed mental subnormals (Eayrs et al., 1993). The implication of this kind of work is that changing the ways in which language and culture construct disability should be regarded as a weapon in the battle for equality (Harpur, 2012), that changes in social attitudes can be initiated by terminological modification.

But in the late twentieth century the usefulness of this linguistic weaponry was sometimes questioned. There was doubt that new terminology could be effective until positive attitudes had improved, for without that change the prejudicial meanings would have become reattached to the liberalised vocabulary (Kirtley, 1975). In fact, an exploration of cross-cultural and historical attitudes toward learning difficulties in Pakistan noted that even where terminology had changed and been made 'non-discriminatory', the attitudes underlying earlier terms surfaced in stigmatising or patronising behaviour (Miles, 1992). These findings clearly problematise the idea that changes in terminology can facilitate changes in attitudes but, judging by a number of probing works (Barnes, 1993; Oliver, 1996; Lunsford, 2006; Rodas, 2009; Vidali, 2010; Bolt, 2014), this is not a dominant criticism within disability studies.

If there is general agreement that the development of language is a prerequisite for changing social attitudes, there is less on precisely what terms are preferable – as is demonstrable in the present book. In the United States and Canada, among other places, the term *people with disabilities* is often endorsed as part of a person-first response to social attitudes that define someone by her or his impairment (Shakespeare, 2006). However, such references to people *with* disabilities are problematic for proponents of the British social model, whereby the person may be impaired but it is only by society that he or she becomes disabled (Barnes and Mercer, 2003; Shakespeare, 2006). Indeed, there are mixed feelings globally about usage of the very word *disability*. For instance, in India, the term *inconvenience* has been used to reduce the negative attitudes that are attached to *impairment* and *disability* (Rao, 2001); while in Japan, past terminology has been recognised as discriminatory and has given way to equivalents of English terms that refer to handicap and disability (Valentine, 2002). The trouble is that the language we use is fundamentally ableist, if not disablist, for the terms *impairment* and *disability* denote deficit in spite of new meanings defined by activists and academics.

This issue may be illustrated with reference to what, in accordance with the preferred language of self-advocacy in the United Kingdom (Nunkoosing and Haydon-Laurelut, 2011), many of us have come to call learning difficulties. In some quarters, this term, like *mental handicap, intellectual disability, intellectual impairment*, and so on, has been superseded by *learning disability*. Certainly, if we consider the usage of these terms in *Disability and Society*, *learning disability* is now the most frequent, having more than doubled since the turn of the century, while *mental handicap* has quartered. However, though often adopted as the choice of professionals (Nunkoosing and Haydon-Laurelut, 2011), the term *learning disability* remains problematic insofar as many people to whom it is attached do not identify as disabled (Inglis, 2013). That is to say, contrary to the ethos of disability pride (Harrison, 1995), for many people the very ascription of the term *learning disabled* constitutes disablism.

Though fundamental, language is only one aspect of the culture by which society is defined. With reference to advertising, for example, the link between attitudes and societal ideologies has been identified by a number of researchers (Hunt, 1966; Brolley and Anderson, 1986; Barnes, 1991; Panol and McBride, 2001). In one study, in order to expand on the hypothesis that attitudes toward people with learning difficulties were negatively influenced by charity advertisements, researchers showed a group of school children two MENCAP posters: one from the 1980s, the other from the 1990s (Doddington et al., 1994). The children who saw the older poster – which was printed in black and white and contrasted the prospects of two boys by asserting that one was going to university, while the other was going nowhere – were more likely to report that it made them feel pity and guilt, and less likely to agree that people with learning difficulties were able to care for themselves. Notably, on seeing this much-criticised poster (Miller et al., 1993;

Eayrs et al., 1994), the school children did not depart significantly on how likely they would be to donate money to the charity, the implication being that the use of more positive imagery would not have discouraged donation (Doddington et al., 1994). That is to say, the negative representation served only to elicit negative attitudes; it contributed to ableism in its laudatory enforcement of normalcy and to disablism in its pejorative representation of impairment.

Although ableism and disablism generally work to a binary logic, whereby people are either disabled or not disabled, a hierarchy of impairments often becomes apparent in social attitudes toward disability. For example, the British Social Attitudes Survey (2005) suggests that people are generally more comfortable with the idea of having a person who is disabled as a neighbour than as a boss or in-law, and that these negative attitudes are especially strong toward people who have so-called mental health problems (Robinson et al., 2007). These findings echo a comparative study in which Israeli students endorsed empowerment and perceived the similarity of people who were disabled to themselves more than they agreed with the prospect of segregation from the community, but were more likely to endorse the exclusion of people who had mental health problems than that of people with learning difficulties – as though the latter were more different and thus less threatening than the former (Schwartz and Armony-Sivan, 2001). What is more, research has found that people who are disabled also hold differing strengths of attitudes toward different impairment groups (Deal, 2003). That is to say, ableism and disablism have resulted in a hierarchy of impairments maintained by people who are disabled and people who are not disabled alike, meaning that problematic attitudes toward disability have made a profound impression in the cultural imagination.

Anomalous practice

Anomalous practice, as noted at the start of this introduction, may be said to demonstrate the profundity of problematic social attitudes toward disability. There is sometimes an assumption that policy and legislation are accompanied or else rapidly followed by social change. After all, in the United States, the United Kingdom, and the Scandinavian countries, by the end of the twentieth century the parent movement for inclusion had succeeded in changing laws, regulations, and funding systems to open the doors of so-called regular schools to many children who were disabled (de Boer et al., 2010). In these terms, the idea is that policies and legislation for social change are put into place and a less disablist ethos soon becomes embedded in the popular imagination, or put differently, becomes part of the 'hegemony', the common-sense understanding of the world (Hyland, 1987). Yet recent history has shown that this is not always the case. In the United Kingdom, at the end of the twentieth century, one in eight of the population was classed as disabled but, despite the Disability Discrimination Act of 1995, services and facilities were still not generally accessible (Chamberlaina, 1998). Accordingly, although the health service had published guidelines on employment in hospitals, workers who were disabled remained conspicuous by their absence

(Chamberlaina, 1998). People who were disabled represented a similarly significant minority population in the United States and also remained underrepresented in the workforce, despite the passage of the Americans with Disabilities Act in 1990 (Hunt and Hunt, 2004). Indeed, given that the impact of legislation in relation to disability has been comparably troubled in, among other places, India (Cobley, 2013), Israel (Soffer et al., 2010), Korea (Kim and Fox, 2011), Sierra Leone (Berghs, 2010), and Turkey (Bezmez and Yardmc, 2010), anomalous practice is evidently an international issue.

That anomalous practice remains so widespread warrants discussion in itself, but it is also important to consider historical details, to explore how the circumstances and experiences of people who are disabled have changed over time in relation to policy and legislation (Purdam et al., 2008). The thing is that policy makers within organisations are influenced by a variety of social factors, as evidenced by, say, the British Scout Association's documented changing attitudes toward disability in the twentieth century. After all, when national policies promoted segregation, during the interwar period, the apparently progressive association encouraged the integration of scouts who were disabled; yet in 1959, when segregative legislation was abolished, the policy of the Scout Association paradoxically changed to exclude people who had learning difficulties from full membership (Stevens, 1995). This historical detail illustrates how progressive legislation may be trumped by disablist policy.

Several important reasons for anomalous practice have been identified. In the United Kingdom, in the case of the Scout Association, the adoption of medical classifications seemed to justify the disablist action (Stevens, 1995), while in the instance of the DDA, a major shortfall was that initially there was no enforcement agency to monitor the implementation (Barnes and Mercer, 2003). What I want us to focus on here, however, is the interrelated point that, in the United States, despite the ADA, potential employers and co-workers maintained negative attitudes toward disability that obstructed progress (Hunt and Hunt, 2004). In fact, a number of case studies gathered at the turn of the century showed that people who were disabled remained vulnerable to disproportionate and complex levels of abuse that were fostered by social attitudes (Calderbank, 2000). The salient point is that, even after legislation, environmental barriers continue to exist, the ultimate and most pervasive being attitudinal (DeJong and Lifchez, 1983). What is more, these social attitudes are rooted in a lack of knowledge and the perpetuation of erroneous stereotypes (Hunt and Hunt, 2004), meaning they can be effortlessly maintained behind the backs of people who are disabled.

The catch is that the presence of people who are disabled has long since been recognised as the key to changing ableist and disablist attitudes. In the late twentieth century, for example, volunteers and people with learning difficulties at the so-called Special Olympics demonstrated that contact contributed to positive changes in attitudes (Roper, 1990). This historical example resonates with the case of hospitals in the United Kingdom, for an obvious but nonetheless important point made by The Royal College of Physicians was that the presence of people who were disabled would have altered attitudes, as had already been found in schools (Chamberlaina, 1998). Indeed, some parents of children who are not disabled have positive attitudes toward inclusive education precisely because they consider it an opportunity to experience the social acceptance of difference (de Boer et al., 2010). The trouble is that from these and other such examples it also follows that, in the absence of contact between people who are and people who are not disabled, attitudes are unlikely to change for the better. Contact may well be a key to change but in its absence, as the present book illustrates, ableist and disablist attitudes are sustained and embellished in many ways.

Overview

The first part of the book illustrates the fact that, though often neglected, an historical analysis of changing social attitudes toward disability is an important area of study (Stevens, 1995). David Doat's opening chapter on prehistory revisits Darwinism by proposing a departure from self-sufficiency and individual capabilities in favour of vulnerability, incompleteness, and interdependence as key conditions of social, moral, and cultural development. Alex Tankard points to the Wild West to show how the reputation of gunfighter Doc Holliday reflects changing attitudes toward tuberculosis and disability over several generations, before Emmeline Burdett ponders one of the lowest points in human history and considers the dehumanising attitudes of the Nazi extermination programme. Alice Hall brings the focus to more recent history and explores the work of two photojournalists injured in Afghanistan, Giles Duley and João Silva, as a challenge to attitudes toward physical impairment in terms of agency, empathy, and everyday experience. In a similarly contemporary vein, Catherine Prendergast's chapter closes the first part of the book with a memoir-informed examination of attitudes toward antipsychotic drugs.

One of the things that becomes evident is the fact that an emancipatory disability research agenda should not avoid the cultural artefacts through which social values and attitudes are shared. I say this because representational methodologies can be utilised in many creative ways that further understandings of changing social attitudes. On a fairly basic level, one past study has found that reading about an encounter with someone who is disabled gives rise to more negative emotions than reading about a similar encounter with someone who is not disabled (Vilchinsky et al., 2010). This capacity to influence social attitudes reveals the importance of critical engagement with representations of disability as a means of change. Research into attitudes toward disability and British television, for example, has resulted in guidelines for programme makers about the importance of disabled people being at the heart of the creative process in order to produce accurate representations and aspiring role models; about breaking down non-disabled viewers' barriers to acceptance; and about disability being less appreciated, as a political concern, than ethnicity or gender (Sancho, 2003). Representational methodologies can be used to interrogate cultural artefacts for manifestations of ableist and disablist attitudes that must be challenged and changed. For these reasons, the second part of the book focuses on the power of cultural representation, the hegemonic potential for influencing social attitudes toward disability. Two of the chapters are concerned with attitudes toward physical impairment, for Tom Coogan explores the cultural history of the so-called hunchback figure and Sue Smith reads a strand of American science fiction literature that features the technological augmentation of the wounded hero. Stella Bolaki's chapter returns the focus of the book to mental health problems with reference to life narratives about schizophrenia – specifically, a memoir by Patrick and Henry Cockburn. The Anglo-American bias of literary disability studies is then challenged as Pauline Eyre encourages us to revisit a novel by Libuše Moníková for its rich and revealing representations of disability. My own chapter sustains the literary focus but juxtaposes it with work on advertising in order to explore assumptions about aesthetics and attitudes toward visual impairment.

The third part of the book reflects the vital role that education plays in creating the social setting by which attitudes are framed (Hyland, 1987). After all, despite the often troubling place of mental health problems in the cultural imagination, purpose-designed education programs have been found to have positive effects on some attitudes toward schizophrenia (Holmes et al., 1999). Along similar lines, in another study, student teachers were surveyed at the start and end of a course on Human Development, which combined formal instruction with fieldwork that involved interviewing members of the community about Down's syndrome and inclusive education, and was found to change attitudes toward disability in general (Campbell and Gilmore, 2003). The present book, however, takes a far more critical approach to education. Alan Hodkinson goes so far as to render the lack of disability in school intranet sites as an ethnic cleansing of space. These concerns about avoidance resonate in Claire Penketh's chapter as she interrogates attitudes toward Special Educational Needs and disability within contemporary art education. Similarly critical of the construct of Special Educational Needs, Owen Barden appropriates the mock learning disability dysrationalia to explain institutional attitudes toward disability, before Craig Collinson focuses on changing attitudes toward dyslexia – a shift from supposed stupidity to designated disability. Finally, Marie Caslin's chapter contends that a change in social attitudes is not desirable but essential because, within the confines of the current British education system, there is no space for pupils labelled with Behavioural, Emotional, and Social Difficulties.

In concluding this introductory chapter it is worth emphasising the premise of the book. Education may be thought of as a profound familiarisation with culture, and it is sometimes said that culture is the glue that holds society together. An exploration of changing social attitudes toward disability, therefore, must take not only the more traditional historical approach to disability studies, but also cultural and educational approaches. Accordingly, the book has a tripartite structure that now moves the main focus through historical, cultural, and educational studies. The multidisciplinarity of this structure is enhanced by the interdisciplinary content of the individual chapters and contributes to the overarching argument that, in relation to disability, changing social attitudes must not be underestimated: they must be critically documented and actively endorsed. Of course we realise that a change in attitudes toward disability may not be sufficient, but nonetheless believe it is a necessary condition of social equality.

References

Barnes, C. (1991) Discrimination: disabled people and the media, *Contact*, 70, 45–48.

Barnes, C. (1993) Political correctness, language and rights, *Rights Not Charity*, 1, 3, 8.

Barnes, C. (2003) What a difference a decade makes: reflections on doing emancipatory' disability research, *Disability and Society*, 18, 1, 3–17.

Barnes, C. and Mercer, G. (2003) *Disability*, Cambridge: Polity.

Berghs, M. (2010) Coming to terms with inequality and exploitation in an African state: researching disability in Sierra Leone, *Disability and Society*, 25, 7, 861–65.

Bezmez, D. and Yardmc, S. (2010) In search of disability rights: citizenship and Turkish disability organizations, *Disability and Society*, 25, 5, 603–15.

Bolt, D. (2014) *The Metanarrative of Blindness: A Re-reading of Twentieth-century Anglophone Writing*, Ann Arbor: University of Michigan Press.

Bolt, D., Rodas, J.M., and Donaldson, E.J. (eds) (2012) *The Madwoman and the Blindman: Jane Eyre, Discourse, Disability*, Columbus: Ohio State University Press.

Brolley, D. and Anderson, S. (1986) Advertising and attitudes, in M. Nagler (ed.) *Perspectives on Disability*, Palo Alto: Health Markets Research.

Calderbank, R. (2000) Abuse and disabled people: vulnerability or social indifference? *Disability and Society*, 15, 3, 521–34.

Campbell, J. and Gilmore, L. (2003) Changing student teachers' attitudes towards disability and inclusion, *Journal of Intellectual and Developmental Disability*, 28, 4, 369–79.

Campbell, F. (2008) Exploring internalised ableism using critical race theory, *Disability and Society*, 23, 2, 151–62.

Cobley, D.S. (2013) Towards economic participation: examining the impact of the convention on the rights of persons with disabilities in India, *Disability and Society*, 28, 4, 441–55.

Chamberlaina, M.A. (1998) Changing attitudes to disability in hospitals, *The Lancet*, 351, 9105, 771–72.

Davis, L.J. (1995) *Enforcing Normalcy: Disability, Deafness and the Body*, London: Verso.

Deal, M. (2003) Disabled people's attitudes toward other impairment groups: a hierarchy of impairments, *Disability and Society*, 18, 7, 897–10.

Deal, M. (2007) Aversive disablism: subtle prejudice toward disabled people, *Disability and Society*, 22, 1, 93–107.

de Boer, A., Pijl, S.J., and Minnaert, A. (2010) Attitudes of parents towards inclusive education: a review of the literature, *European Journal of Special Needs Education*, 25, 2, 165–81.

DeJong, G. and Lifchez, R. (1983) Physical disability and public policy, *Scientific American*, 248, 6, 40–49.

Doddington, K., Jones, R.S.P., and Miller, B.Y. (1994) Are attitudes to people with learning disabilities negatively influenced by charity advertising? *Disability and Society*, 9, 2, 207–22.

Eayrs, C.B., Ellis, N., Jones, R.S.P., and Miller, B.Y. (1994) Representations of learning disability in the literature of charity campaigns, in I. Markova and R. Farr (eds) *Representations of Health, Illness and Handicap*, New York: Harwood Academic.

Eayrs, C.B., Ellis, N., and Jones, R.S.P. (1993) Which label? An investigation into the effects of terminology on public perceptions of and attitudes towards people with learning difficulties, *Disability, Handicap and Society*, 8, 2, 111–27.

Finkelstein, V. (1980) *Attitudes and Disabled People*, Washington: World Rehabilitation Fund.

Harpur, P. (2012) From disability to ability: changing the phrasing of the Debate, *Disability and Society*, 27, 3, 325–37.

Harrison, T. (1995) *Disability: Rights and Wrongs*, Oxford: Lion.

Holmes, P., Corrigan, P.W., Williams, P., Conor, J., and Kubiak, M.A. (1999) Changing attitudes about schizophrenia, *Schizophrenia Bulletin*, 25, 3, 447–56.

Hunt, C.S. and Hunt, B. (2004) Changing attitudes toward people with disabilities experimenting with an educational intervention, *Journal of Managerial Issues*, 16, 2, 266–80.

Hunt, P. (1966) *Stigma: The Experience of Disability*, London: Geoffrey Chapman.

Hyland, T. (1987) Disability and the moral point of view, *Disability, Handicap and Society*, 2, 2, 163–73.

Inglis, P.A. (2013) Reinterpreting learning difficulty: a professional and personal challenge? *Disability and Society*, 28, 3, 423–26.

Isaac, R., Raja, B.W.D., and Ravanan, M.P. (2010) Integrating people with disabilities: their right – our responsibility, *Disability and Society*, 25, 5, 627–30.

Kim, K.M. and Fox, M.H. (2011) A comparative examination of disability anti-discrimination legislation in the United States and Korea, *Disability and Society*, 26, 3, 269–83.

Kirtley, D.D. (1975) *The Psychology of Blindness*, Chicago: Nelson-Hall.

Lunsford, S. (2006) The debate within: authority and the discourse of blindness, *Journal of Visual Impairment and Blindness*, 100, 1, 26–35.

The National Centre for Social Research (2005) *The British Social Attitudes Survey*, London: The National Centre for Social Research.

Madriaga, M. (2007) Enduring disablism: students with dyslexia and their pathways into UK higher education and beyond, *Disability and Society*, 22, 4, 399–412.

Miles, M. (1992) Concepts of mental retardation in Pakistan: toward cross-cultural and historical perspectives, *Disability, Handicap and Society*, 7, 3, 235–55.

Miller, B.Y., Jones, R.S.P., and Ellis, N. (1993) Group differences in response to charity images of children with Down's Syndrome, *Down's Syndrome Research and Practice*, 1, 118–22.

Nunkoosing, K. and Haydon-Laurelut, M. (2011) Intellectual disabilities, challenging behaviour and referral texts: a critical discourse analysis, *Disability and Society*, 26, 4, 405–17.

Oliver, M. (1992) Changing the social relations of research production? *Disability, Handicap and Society*, 7, 2, 101–14.

Oliver, M. (1996) Defining impairment and disability: issues at stake, in C. Barnes and G. Mercer (eds) *Exploring the Divide: Chronic Illness and Disability*, Leeds: Disability Press.

Panol, Z.S. and McBride, M. (2001) Disability images in print advertising: exploring attitudinal impact issues, *Disability Studies Quarterly*, 21.

Purdam, K., Afkhami, R., Olsen, W., and Thornton, P. (2008) Disability in the UK: measuring equality, *Disability and Society*, 23, 1, 53–65.

Rao, S. (2001) A little inconvenience: perspectives of Bengali families of children with disabilities on labelling and inclusion, *Disability and Society*, 16, 4, 531–48.

Robinson, C., Martin, J., and Thompson, K. (2007) *Attitudes towards and Perceptions of Disabled People – Findings from a Module Included in the 2005 British Social Attitudes Survey*, Disability Rights Commission.

Rodas, J.M. (2009) On blindness, *Journal of Literary and Cultural Disability Studies*, 3, 2, 115–30.

Roper, P. (1990) Changing perceptions through contact, disability, *Handicap and Society*, 5, 3, 243–55.

Sancho, J. (2003) *Disabling Prejudice Attitudes towards Disability and its Portrayal on Television*, London: British Broadcasting Corporation, the Broadcasting Standards Commission and the Independent Television Commission.

Schwartz, C. and Armony-Sivan, R. (2001) Students' attitudes to the inclusion of people with disabilities in the community, *Disability and Society*, 16, 3, 403–13.

Shakespeare, T. (2006) *Disability Rights and Wrongs*, Oxon: Routledge.

Snyder, S.L. and Mitchell, D.T. (2006) *Cultural Locations of Disability*, Chicago: University of Chicago Press.

Söder, M. (1990) Prejudice or ambivalence? Attitudes toward persons with disabilities, *Disability, Handicap and Society*, 5, 3, 227–41.

Soffer, M., Rimmerman, A., Blanck, P., and Hill, E. (2010) Media and the Israeli disability rights legislation: progress or mixed and contradictory images? *Disability and Society*, 25, 6, 687–99.

Stevens, A. (1995) Changing attitudes to disabled people in the Scout Association in Britain (1908–62): a contribution to a history of disability, *Disability and Society*, 10, 3, 281–94.

Thomas, C. (2004) How is disability understood? An examination of sociological approaches, *Disability and Society*, 19, 6, 569–83.

Tregaskis, C. (2000) Interviewing non-disabled people about their disability-related attitudes: seeking methodologies, *Disability and Society*, 15, 2, 343–53.

Valentine, J. (2002) Naming and narrating disability in Japan, in M. Corker and T. Shakespeare (eds) *Disability/Postmodernity: Embodying Disability Theory*, London: Continuum.

Vidali, A. (2010) Seeing what we know: disability and theories of metaphor, *Journal of Literary and Cultural Disability Studies*, 4, 1, 33–54.

Vilchinsky, N., Findler, L., and Werner, S. (2010) Attitudes toward people with disabilities: the perspective of attachment theory, *Rehabilitation Psychology*, 55, 3, 298–306.

Part I
Disability, attitudes, and history

1 Evolution and human uniqueness

Prehistory, disability, and the unexpected anthropology of Charles Darwin

David Doat

There is an ableist anthropology that underlies most scientific work on evolutionary theories, one that states that vulnerability and disability have neither function nor positive meaning in the evolutionary process of our species. This is a tacit reason why such thematics are often either left out of conversations by evolutionnists or limited to the controversial issues raised by eugenics. It also implies inappropriate behaviours and attitudes toward disability. In this chapter, I suggest that we should reread the writings of Charles Darwin, for contrary to strong social beliefs among contemporary scientific communities, the founder of the theory of natural selection was neither a strong defender of eugenics nor a social Darwinist. I conclude by insisting upon the legitimacy of a new interdisciplinary research field that focuses on the survival of disabled members in prehistoric human groups. Because ableism conditions modern narratives that have been written about the past (Finlay, 1999), it is only by focusing on new philosophical, scientific, and (pre)historical research that the history of human evolution may appear less ableist.

The ableist anthropology that underlies scientific discourses

We may well be convinced by modern accounts of human evolution (Huxley, 1941; Dobzhansky, 1962; Jones et al., 1994; Mayr, 2001; Dunbar, 2004), especially educational accounts that focus on language, mastering the environment through technology, and the development of human intelligence (Potts et al., 2010; Roberts, 2011). Nevertheless, many of these accounts spread an incomplete vision of humanity, for they do not take into consideration the universal facts of vulnerability and disability.

Because some members of our species are affected by loss of 'normal powers' due to disability, they appear marginal and unnecessary in developing the highest human faculties that contribute to the evolutionary success of human beings. Vulnerability and disability seem to be devoid of meaning in most contemporary scientific accounts of human evolution. At best, they are interpreted as the price to be paid in a 'nasty and brutish' evolutionary process based on natural selection, survival of the fittest, suffering, and a high death toll (Monod, 1974; Dawkins,

2006). From this perspective, it seems difficult to demonstrate in an evolutionary framework (whereby utility function is essential) the 'value' of a 'severely' disabled individual. As a corollary, eugenics and human enhancement appear to be the only answers to disability. This is the obvious conclusion, unless the interpretation that disabled individuals do not have a contributory role to play in the development of human ontology is recognised as the result of an ableist (i.e., culturally and historically limited) vision of human beings.

What occurs in economic and political fields of academic research – as has already been highlighted (Kittay, 1999; Nussbaum, 2006) – also happens in biological and evolutionary ones: humans are generally seen as independent agents. The pictures of the Past that evolutionists reconstruct remain essentially ableist in character (Finlay, 1999; Le Pichon, 2007). Human relationships are systematically based on a prescriptive understanding of an autonomous human being, driven by *rational interests*, and possessing all *cognitive* and *physical faculties*. Indeed, this is an anthropological assumption that is theoretically required (e.g., in evolutionary ethics and game theory) to make sense of both selfish and altruistic behaviours in the scope of mathematic and economic modelling (Sober and Wilson, 1999; Bowles and Gintis, 2013). In this type of modelling of human sociality, it is difficult to find a place for persons experiencing social dependency on a daily basis. Altruism is always interpreted as occurring between fully 'self-supportive' individuals (or groups of individuals) capable of struggling to survive.

Under this anthropological bias, the characteristics of human beings as always vulnerable and sometimes disabled are never taken into account. Instead we try to hold onto ableist models that produce the 'best' theoretical results. By excluding human vulnerability and disability from anthropological and evolutionary concerns, some scholars (Rachels, 1991; Singer, 2011) build their scientific and ethical theories on the philosophical pretence that humans are *ontologically* independent (i.e., that the cooperation between persons that some insist is *inter*dependence is simply mutual and voluntary cooperation between *a priori* independent rational individuals).

A fresh look at the works of Charles Darwin: are humans like gorillas?

Because of modern dominant accounts of human evolution and the underlying philosophical anthropology they reflect, human fragility and disability have been left out of the elements that have played a significant and decisive role in our evolutionary history. As the nineteenth- and twentieth-century interest in the concept of 'degeneration' demonstrates, the scientific community used to think that the lack of adaptive skills in some individuals might even interfere with the progressive development of a human society in complete and full control of its destiny. It was in reaction to this fear that many eugenic policies based on the theories of Darwin were born in the nineteenth century (Stiker, 1999). Yet the founder of modern biology did not fully subscribe to all of these theories. Although he was influenced by the bourgeois-liberal culture of his time, the 'concrete suggestions for encouraging reproduction of the valuable members of society or discouraging it by the undesirable members seemed to Darwin either impractical or morally suspect' (Paul, 2003: 223). Furthermore, judging by his anthropological assumptions, he was aware of the frailty of humanity and of the nature relative to the very concepts of 'weakness', 'force', 'ability', and so on (Tort, 2001; Paul and Moore, 2010). Contrary to eugenicists of his time, then, Darwin had both philosophical and scientific reasons to believe that 'caring' for disabled members was neither senseless nor disadvantageous in human groups.

Fundamentally, Darwin's philosophical anthropology, which is *implicit* in his scientific writings, differs from that of the theorists of social Darwinism, eugenics, and socio-biology. Although Francis Galton, the founder of eugenics, was Darwin's cousin, neither private letters nor public writings demonstrated that Darwin *fully* adhered to his cousin's ideas (Tort, 2008). This is because the anthropology of Darwin takes into account the vulnerability of the human subject. Rather than insisting on individual autonomy, Darwin developed a 'community selection' theory (Richards, 2003: 101-109) of the sociocognitive development and moral sense of humans. This theory relies on a keen awareness of human vulnerability and the relational processes that contribute to balance in the interdependency relationships that characterise human societies.

Twelve years after *On the Origin of Species*, Darwin claimed in *The Descent of Man* that human beings could not have developed their most admirable mental abilities without the 'fragility' characteristic to their organic form. Wondering whether he should not have descended from a gorilla or a smaller and less independent species of ape, Darwin wrote in *The Descent of Man*:

> In regard to bodily size or strength, we do not know whether man is descended from some small species, like the chimpanzee, or from one as powerful as the gorilla; and, therefore, we cannot say whether man has become larger and stronger, or smaller and weaker, than his ancestors. We should, however, bear in mind that an animal possessing great size, strength, and ferocity, and which, like the gorilla, could defend itself from all enemies, would not perhaps have become social: and this would most effectually have checked the acquirement of the higher mental qualities, such as sympathy and the love of his fellows. Hence it might have been an immense advantage to man to have sprung from some comparatively weak creature. The small strength and speed of man, his want of natural weapons, etc., are more than counterbalanced, firstly, by his intellectual powers, through which he has formed for himself weapons, tools, etc., though still remaining in a barbarous state, and, secondly, by his social qualities which lead him to give and receive aid from his fellow-man.
>
> (Darwin, 1874: 63–64)

Patrick Tort, a specialist in Darwin's works in France, highlights that Darwin observed that the individual strength of a gorilla, its ability to defend itself, represented an obstacle for socialisation and that a similar disposition in the human subject would have checked the acquisition of the highest mental qualities (Tort, 2008). Human vulnerability appears as a selected advantage that calls for union in the face of danger; it calls for cooperation and mutual aid (Tort, 2008); and it contributes to the correlative development of intelligence by assuming the protection of people who cannot defend themselves. In other words, for Darwin, our evolutionary victory is not solely dependent on higher cognitive abilities, culture, technology or language. It also appears necessarily linked to our vulnerability, interdependency, and inclination for social care, which have consistently pushed humanity to compensate by relying more on what is cultural, technological, and symbolic (Finkelstein, 1998: 28).

John Dewey, one of the founders of pragmatism, proposed an interesting evolutionary take on this subject:

> We may imagine a leader in an early social group, when the question had arisen of putting to death the feeble, the sickly, and the aged, in order to give that group an advantage in the struggle for existence with other groups; – we may imagine him, I say, speaking as follows: 'No. In order that we may secure this advantage, let us preserve these classes [whether disabled or not]. It is true for the moment that they make an additional drain upon our resources, and an additional tax upon the energies which might otherwise be engaged in fighting our foes. But in looking after these helpless we shall develop habits of foresight and forethought, powers of looking before and after, tendencies to husband our means, which shall ultimately make us the most skilled in warfare. We shall foster habits of group loyalty, feelings of solidarity, which shall bind us together by such close ties that no social group which has not cultivated like feelings through caring for all its members, will be able to withstand us'. In a word, such conduct would pay in the struggle for existence as well as be morally commendable. If the group to which he spoke saw any way to tide over the immediate emergency, no one can gainsay the logic of this speech. Not only the prolongation of the period of dependence, but the multiplication of its forms, has meant historically increase of intelligent foresight and planning, and increase of the bonds of social unity. Who shall say that such qualities are not positive instruments in the struggle for existence, and that those who stimulate and call out such powers are not among those 'fit to survive'?
>
> (Dewey, 1898: 326)

Here, the 'less able' coincides with the human who does not make paying attention to human vulnerability, interdependence, and mutual *caring practices* central in her or his life. The concept of 'care' to which I refer does not assume that any relations between care receivers and care providers are asymmetric (and paternalistic). As David Bolt writes, 'While there is a received understanding that disabled people are dependent on non-disabled people, the reverse is frequently unacknowledged but also true, as has been portrayed in many works of fiction that blur the distinction between non-disabled care-provider and disabled dependant' (Bolt, 2008: para. 11). On the other hand, 'caring practices' must be distinguished from 'curing practices', for they do not (only) refer to the medical field. Indeed, parenting, socio-educational development, professional activities, religious and cultural commitments, political affairs, friendship, and so on, imply different relationships of care among humans. More broadly, care is a corporeal potential that involves meeting the needs and maintaining the world of our self and others. It is 'committed to the flourishing and growth of individuals yet acknowledges our interconnectedness and interdependence' (Hamington, 2004: 3). Care could yet be defined as a human practice that includes 'everything we do to help individuals to meet their ... needs, develop or maintain their ... capabilities, and avoid or alleviate unnecessary or unwanted pain and suffering, so that they can survive, develop, and function in society' (Engster, 2007: 28).

Contrary to eugenic theories, a fresh reading of Darwin's anthropology contradicts the idea that society only evolves through the elimination of its most vulnerable members. Indeed, it is not only our strength but also our limitations and incompleteness that we must take on in evolution, for it is a relational and rational form of *compensation* for our fragility that makes us unique. This anthropological hypothesis (see Finkelstein, 1998) is one of the reasons why Darwin could state:

> We civilised men ... do our utmost to check the process of elimination; we build asylums for the imbecile, the maimed, and the sick; we institute poor-laws; and our medical men exert their utmost skill to save the life of every one to the last moment.
>
> (Darwin, 1874: 133)

This 'medical' and somewhat 'paternalist' vocabulary is outmoded, but what remains important is the dysgenic claim (Tort, 2008: 86) of the founder of modern biology. Indeed, in accordance with factors that, for him, prevailed throughout human development, Darwin added:

> We must therefore bear the undoubtedly bad effects of the weak surviving and propagating their kind [Darwin is referring to the notion held by eugenic theories of the 'degeneration' of the species], for 'Nor could we check our sympathy [i.e., for people who are disabled], even at the urging of hard reason [in relation to the economy], without deterioration in the noblest part of our nature'.
>
> (Darwin, 1874: 134)

Here, the 'noblest part of our nature' refers to the *vulnerable* and *unaccomplished* form (i.e., the 'essence') of the human being, along with behaviours of sympathy and care that are required, at any moment, by the inherent humanity of the human subject. This is why the apparently incomplete and fragile body of a disabled person has a major ethical and ontological force that is both revealing and full of symbolic meaning in the history of all human cultures.

In this 'inclusive' vision of humanity, there is no longer a legitimate gap between vulnerable beings (who could be denounced as such because of a disability) and strong individuals (both disabled and non-disabled). This dichotomy, which led to some eugenic policies in the nineteenth and twentieth centuries, comes to light when the modern, functional, and autonomous subject forgets that her or his real strength has its roots in vulnerability and openness:

> Far from being a burden our imperfections in relation to other animals might be regarded as one of the essential characteristics that make us human. In this respect disabled people are the most human of beings. The segregation of disabled people from our non-disabled peers, then, is not only an inhuman event ... but the hiatus between specialist knowledge confined to 'disablement' and public knowledge concerned with 'normality' is no less than the emergence of a profoundly disabling pedagogical barrier in the evolution of human understanding.
>
> (Finkelstein, 1998: 29)

In other words, if we want to develop a better understanding of the evolutionary processes that are specifically involved in human sociality, we are required to deal with the classical assumption that the vast majority of a population are productive, invulnerable, and self-sufficient most of the time (Dettwyler, 1991). Not only does this imply that dependency and weakness are the only characteristics of some 'marginal' categories of persons in human communities, it is also another formulation of the ideological reductionism of human complexity into two fixed groups: the non-disabled and the disabled, the strong and the weak, the productive and the non-productive, the independent and the vulnerable, and so on. Because of such ideological divisions, studies published in the twentieth century by evolutionists who insisted on the importance of tools, language, or large brains to define 'human uniqueness', often assumed the common stereotype of modern western society, that disabled people cannot contribute to society. For such scientists (Solecki, 1971; Gould, 1988; Trinkaus and Shipman, 1993; Vilos, 2011; Gorman, 2012), disabled people only survived because of the compassion of nondisabled members in human groups.

Contrary to such a view, postmodernist approaches like disability studies, feminist studies, and care studies (see Finkelstein, 1998; Kittay, 1999; Hamington, 2004) recognise that the continuum of dependency in human groups always points to a 'middle ground', to 'the fact that the extremes of parasitic dependency and independence are both myths' (Bolt, 2014: 65), for there is an anthropological continuity between the least and most dependent individuals in human groups. In other words, we have to rebalance the classical assumption, as every population has members who are occasionally, temporarily, or permanently disabled. Consequently, social interdependence and care are omnipresent facts of humanity.

For Tom Shakespeare, this was particularly true in prehistoric populations: 'Exigencies of life may have rendered more people impaired ... disfigurement and limitation was a fact of life "nasty, brutish and short". Therefore our notions of the division between "able-bodied" and "disabled" may need to be revised' (Shakespeare, 1999: 101). They have to be revised, for instance, from the point of view of a philosophical anthropology that needs to be much more inclusive than the one that many contemporary evolutionists still assume.

Archaeological and paleopathological discoveries: a new look at human evolution

An interest in conditions for disabled people in prehistory has begun to emerge with archaeological and paleopathological progress (Finlay, 1999). This new field of research may be an empirical argument for the 'inclusive' anthropology that I adopt in this chapter, in order to get a better understanding of Darwin's reluctance about eugenics. Indeed, a growing number of remains have been recovered that show paleopathological evidence of impairments (Ortner, 2003) that would have precluded 'normal' functioning, resulting in a disability. Such empirical discoveries unquestionably show that there is a correlation between the emergence of humanity, humanisation, and social care involving symbiotic relations between disabled and non-disabled members of prehistoric human groups.

Among the first clues of such a correlation was the famous discovery by Ralph Solecki (1971) in a cave of the Zagros mountains in Iraq. When Solecki popularised one of the first significant paleopathological findings in his book entitled *Shanidar, The First Flower People*, many scientists expressed strong doubts about his conclusions regarding inclusive attitudes toward disability in Prehistory (Le Pichon, 2009: paragraph 17). Since then, it has been well established (Lebel et al., 2001; Degusta 2002; Tilley and Oxenham, 2011) that caring practices toward disabled people were not an exception in Prehistory (Hublin, 2009). Indeed, through analysis of bones and remains, most archaeologists and paleopathologists argue today that caring practices toward disabled members of hunter-gatherer communities may have existed more than 100,000 years ago (Berkson, 2004). That is to say, although the exclusion of disabled people has characterised social life since before the evolution of *homo sapiens*, inclusive responses that compensate for disability have also been common in human societies.

Paleopathological remains raise questions of primary importance relating to disability in Prehistory, which must be carefully explored by scholars involved in archaeology and disability studies (Southwell-Wright, 2013). As Shakespeare writes:

It is both timely and encouraging that archaeologists have begun to confront the questions posed by the ever-presence of disability, and to interrogate both the practice of archaeology and the historical/prehistorical record. One of the most interesting aspects of this engagement is the role of archaeology on the crossover between the sciences and the humanities. While disability studies has developed in distinction from the dominant medical approaches to disablement, and has largely turned its back on matters of anatomy, physiology and pathology, archaeology has the capacity to revisit and problematize issues of the human body in time, and to connect the physical to the socio-cultural. This offers opportunities, but also dangers.

(Shakespeare, 1999: 99–100)

Indeed, Disability scholars and palopathologists/archaeologists have to face many challenges. In the skeletal record, assessing which 'abnormalities' may be defined as disabling to the individual or to the group in which he or she lived is difficult (Roberts, 1999: 81). As archaeologist Christopher J. Knüsel writes, 'We must be aware that definitions of disability and reactions to disability very likely differed in the past, as well as among different groups in the present' (Knüsel, 1999: 32). It is unlikely, for example, that dyslexia would have been a disability in prehistoric societies. Moreover, because behaviours do not fossilise, there is little empirical data to assess how prehistorical societies behaved toward disability. For instance, caring for disabled people with love or preventing them to die in order to treat them as 'scapegoats' is an alternative that paleopathological data cannot systematically help to clarify (Dettwyler, 1991). Material evidence can 'show the effects of disease or trauma a person experienced, but on its own it cannot show the cultural or social aspects of that person's life conclusively' (Metzler, 1999: 64). Finally, while considering the present may be useful (Roberts, 2013), contemporary researchers may 'impose their ideas upon the past, without considering that concepts and perceptions may have changed considerably through time' (Roberts, 1999: 81). Despite all the challenges, contemporary literature that connects disability to the past can set out 'some of the [most] fascinating problems and paradoxes, and open up a considerable area for further research and scholarship' (Shakespeare, 1999: 101).

Conclusion: transforming social beliefs in scientific communities

Exclusionary behaviours and attitudes toward disability have existed throughout human history and in *all* human societies, which obviously is, and should be, a key focus in disability studies. But when we focus on exclusion, we sometimes risk endorsing a theoretical bias: we may neglect 'natural' (i.e., given) inclusive practices in human groups. For example, we may come to 'take – as given – the ideological and material exclusion of people with labels of physical, sensory or cognitive impairments' (Goodley, 2010: xi). If ableist and disablist attitudes are considered *a priori* as given, however, 'spontaneous' inclusive behaviors among human groups risk being seen *a priori* as improbable, if not impossible. This is why my exploration of prehistorical social attitudes toward disability revisits the work of Darwin. As demonstrated by empirical research in ethology (Silk, 1992; de Waal, 2009; Fashing and Nguyen, 2011), some animal societies are able to organise themselves in order to include and take care of their injured members. Since for Darwin there was neither break nor natural gap between human species and animals, why would the human animal not fall within this 'natural' continuity? Moreover, at a group level it is not contrary to natural selection to assume that developing symbiotic care practices is advantageous in human societies from a Darwinian evolutionary perspective. This claim should increase scientific interest in a new field of research dedicated to disability in Prehistory, for it may be one more stone in the reconstruction of a more balanced (less ableist) history of human origins.

References

Berkson, G. (2004) Intellectual and physical disabilities in prehistory and early civilization, *Mental Retardation*, 42, 3, 195–208.

Bolt, D. (2008) *Symbiosis and Subjectivity: Literary Representations of Disability and Social Care*. Online. Available www.disability-studies.leeds.ac.uk/files/library/bolt-Simbiosis-and-Subjectivity.pdf (accessed 24 September 2013).

Bolt, D. (2014) *The Metanarrative of Blindness: A Re-reading of Twentieth-century Anglophone Writing*, Ann Arbor: University of Michigan Press.

Bowles, S. and Gintis, H. (2013) *A Cooperative Species: Human Reciprocity and Its Evolution*, Princeton: Princeton University Press.

Darwin, C. (1874) *The Descent of Man, and Selection in Relation to Sex*, London: John Murray.

Dawkins, R. (2006) *The Selfish Gene*, Oxford, New York: Oxford University Press.

Degusta, D. (2002) Comparative skeletal pathology and the case for conspecific care in middle Pleistocene Hominids, *Journal of Archaeological Science*, 29, 12, 1435–1438.

Dettwyler, K.A. (1991) Can paleopathology provide evidence for 'compassion'? *American Journal of Physical Anthropology*, 84, 4, 375–384.

de Waal, F.B.M. (2009) *The Age of Empathy: Nature's Lessons for a Kinder Society*, New York: Three Rivers Press.

Dewey, J. (1898) Evolution and ethics, *The Monist*, VIII, 321–341.

Dobzhansky, T. (1962) *Mankind Evolving: The Evolution of the Human Species*, New Haven: Yale University Press.

Dunbar, R.I.M. (2004) *The Human Story*, London: Faber and Faber.

Engster, D. (2007) *The Heart of Justice*, Oxford: Oxford University Press.

Fashing, P.J. and Nguyen, N. (2011) Behavior toward the dying, diseased, or disabled among animals and its relevance to Paleopathology, *International Journal of Paleopathology*, 1, 3–4, 128–129.

Finkelstein, V. (1998) Emancipating disabling studies, in T. Shakespeare (ed.) *The Disability Reader: Social Science Perspectives*, London: Continuum International Publishing Group Ltd.

Finlay, N. (1999) Disability archaeology: an introduction, *Archeological Review from Cambridge*, 15, 2, 1–6.

Goodley, D. (2010) *Disability Studies: An Interdisciplinary Introduction*, London: SAGE.

Gorman, J. (2012) Ancient bones that tell a story of compassion, *The New York Times*. Online. Available www.nytimes.com/2012/12/18/science/ancient-bones-that-tell-a-story-of-compassion.html (accessed 24 September 2013).

Gould, S.J. (1988) Honorable men and women, *Natural History*, 97, 3, 16–20.

Hamington, M. (2004) *Embodied Care: Jane Addams, Maurice Merleau-Ponty, and Feminist Ethics*, Urbana: University of Illinois Press.

Hublin, J.J. (2009) The prehistory of compassion, *Proceedings of the National Academy of Sciences*, 106, 16, 6429–6430.

Huxley, J. (1941) *The Uniqueness of Man*, London: Chatto and Windus.

Jones, S., Martin, R.D., and Pilbeam, D.R. (1994) *The Cambridge Encyclopedia of Human Evolution*, Cambridge, New York: Cambridge University Press.

Kittay, E.F. (1999) *Love's Labor: Essays on Women, Equality, and Dependency*, New York: Routledge.

Knüsel, C.J. (1999) Orthopaedic disability: some hard evidence, *Archaeological Review from Cambridge*, 15, 2, 31–53.

Lebel, S., Trinkaus, E., Faure, M., Fernandez, P., Guerin, C., Richter, D., Mercier, N., Valladas, H., and Wagner, W.A. (2001) Comparative morphology and Paleobiology of middle Pleistocene human remains from the Bau de l'Aubesier, Vaucluse, France, *Proceedings of the National Academy of Sciences*, 98, 20, 11097–11102.

Mayr, E. (2001) *What Evolution Is*, New York: Basic.

Metzler, I. (1999) The Paleopathology of disability in the middle ages, *Archaeological Review from Cambridge*, 15, 2, 55–67.

Monod, J. (1974) *Chance and Necessity*, London: Fontana.

Nussbaum, M.C. (2006) *Frontiers of Justice: Disability, Nationality, Species Membership*, Cambridge: Harvard University Press.

Ortner, D.J. (2003) *Identification of Pathological Disorders in Human Skeletal Remains*, Amsterdam: Academic.

Paul, D.B. (2003) Darwin, social Darwinism and eugenics, in J. Hodge and G. Radick (eds) *The Cambridge Companion to Darwin*, Cambridge: Cambridge University Press.

Paul, D.B. and Moore, J. (2010) The Darwinian context: evolution and inheritance, in A. Bashford and P. Levine (eds) *The Oxford Handbook of the History of Eugenics*, Oxford: Oxford University Press.

Le Pichon, X. (2007) *Aux Racines de l'Homme: de la Mort à l'Amour* [To the roots of man. From death to love], Paris: Presses de la Renaissance.

Le Pichon, X. (2009) Ecce Homo ('Behold Humanity'). *On Being*. Online. Available www. onbeing.org/program/fragility-and-evolution-our-humanity/feature/ecce-homo-behold-humanity/1561 (accessed 24 September 2013).

Potts, R., Sloan, C. and National Museum of Natural History (U.S.) (2010) *What Does It Mean To Be Human?* Washington: National Geographic.

Rachels, J. (1991) *Created from Animals: The Moral Implications of Darwinism*, Oxford: Oxford University Press.

Richards, R.J. (2003) Darwin on minds, morals and emotions, in J. Hodge and G. Radick (eds) *The Cambridge Companion to Darwin*, Cambridge: Cambridge University Press.

Roberts, A.M. (2011) *Evolution: The Human Story*, London: Dorling Kindersley.

Roberts, C. (1999) Disability in the skeletal record: assumptions, problems and some examples, *Archaeological Review from Cambridge*, 15, 2, 79–97.

Roberts, C. (2013) *Bioarchaeology and 'Disability': Using the Present to Inform Interpretations of Past Impairment.* Online. Available www.meeting.physanth.org/program/2013/session43/roberts-2013-bioarchaeology-and-disability-using-the-present-to-inform-interpretations-of-past-impairment.html (accessed 24 September 2013).

Shakespeare, T. (1999) Commentary: observations on disability and archaeology, *Archaeological Review from Cambridge*, 15, 2, 99–101.

Silk, J.B. (1992) The origins of caregiving behavior, *American Journal of Physical Anthropology*, 87, 2, 227–229.

Singer, P. (2011) *The Expanding Circle: Ethics, Evolution, and Moral Progress*, Princeton: Princeton University Press.

Sober, E. and Wilson, D.S. (1999) *Unto Others: The Evolution and Psychology of Unselfish Behavior*, Cambridge: Harvard University Press.

Solecki, R.S. (1971) *Shanidar, The First Flower People*, New York: Knopf.

Southwell-Wright, W. (2013) *Past Perspectives: What Can Archaeology Offer Disability Studies?* Online. Available www.academia.edu/3277906/Past_perspectives_What_can_archaeology_offer_disability_studies (accessed 26 September 2013).

Stiker, H.J. (1999) *A History of Disability*, Ann Arbor: University of Michigan Press.

Tilley, L. and Oxenham, M.F. (2011) Survival against the odds: modeling the social implications of care provision to seriously disabled individuals, *International Journal of Paleopathology*, 1, 1, 35–42.

Tort, P. (2001) *Darwin and the Science of Evolution*, New York: Harry N. Abrams.

Tort, P. (2008) *L'effet Darwin: sélection naturelle et naissance de la civilisation* [The Darwin effect: natural selection and the birth of civilization], Paris: Seuil.

Trinkaus, E. and Shipman, P. (1993) *The Neanderthals: Changing the Image of Mankind*, New York: Knopf.

Vilos, J. (2011) *Bioarchaeology of Compassion: Exploring Extreme Cases of Pathology in a Bronze Age Skeletal Population from Tell Abraq, U.A.E.* Online. Available www. digitalscholarship.unlv.edu/thesesdissertations/967 (accessed 24 September 2013).

2 Killer consumptive in the Wild West

The posthumous decline of Doc Holliday

Alex Tankard

In 1882, journalists in Colorado interviewed the deadliest gunfighter in the Wild West. John Henry 'Doc' Holliday (1851–1887) was a man devoid of fear, reputed to have killed up to fifty men ('Caught in Denver', 1882). Yet journalists were astonished to discover he was also a genteel, frail-looking 'consumptive' living with incurable tuberculosis. Holliday's consumptive body fascinated contemporaries – partly because this impairment was traditionally associated with a Romantic, sentimental disabled identity, quite incongruous with his brutal reputation, and partly because he seemed physically incapable of violence: one journalist even marvelled that his slender wrists could hold a gun ('Awful Arizona', 1882). These early descriptions emphasised above all the elective aspects of his physical presence – his polished manners and exquisite dress and grooming – and presented his consumptive body not as a passive object of pathology or pity but, rather, as an essential component of a persona defined by self-possession, neatness, and 'a suavity of manner for which he was always noted' ('Caught', 1882).

Holliday's contemporaries delighted in the debonair consumptive gunfighter, but this delight did not last long after his death: this chapter focuses on the changing social attitudes toward tuberculosis in particular (and disability in general) that distorted Holliday's reputation in posterity. In the 1900s, the increasing dominance of biomedical models of disability and new public panic about contagion began to overpower traditionally favourable attitudes toward consumptives. The delicate 'consumptive' body became the diseased, distasteful 'tubercular' body. Indeed, of six major film representations of Holliday since 1946, five failed to cast actors who even *looked* consumptive. While Holliday's delicate physique was a crucial (and appealing) aspect of his persona in the 1880s, Hollywood refused to depict it on screen.

One exception to the rule of refusal is Dennis Quaid's portrayal of Holliday in *Wyatt Earp* (1994). Unfortunately, while the presence of a fragile-looking body on screen could offer audiences some insight into Holliday's precarious existence in a violent society, the film squanders this opportunity by ignoring the cultural context of his disability. *Wyatt Earp* insists that the tubercular (no longer 'consumptive') body is unbearable, and overrides any historical evidence that does not fit with this ableist judgement. Ironically, the film's tendency to treat early eye-witness descriptions of Holliday as mistakes in need of ableist correction is the strongest indication that Holliday's disabled identity was unsettling and disruptive for subsequent writers attempting to impose judgements on his life. The 'corrections' expose the aspects of Holliday's persona with most disruptive potential: his confident, elegant self-presentation, his life and death outside biomedical institutions, and his clear assertion that a life with incurable impairment was worth defending.

The consumptive gunfighter before 1900

In the 1880s, Holliday was one of an estimated 200,000 American consumptives ('Talks', 1886: 4), and perhaps one-third of Coloradan settlers were 'health-seekers' (Baur, 1959: 105). Many regions that Holliday visited were popular consumptive health resorts with large – even majority – disabled populations (Rothman, 1995: 3, 132; Roberts, 2006: 103, 160, 369). Tuberculosis played an important part not only in Holliday's story, but also in the story of the American West.

Holliday probably developed tuberculosis, then called 'consumption', 'phthisis' or 'decline', while training as a dentist in the early 1870s. He travelled West from Georgia in 1873 and, as the years went by, drifted further into the violent frontier subculture of professional gamblers (see Courtwright, 1996: 82; 97, on homicide statistics for towns Holliday inhabited). In 1882, his involvement in vigilantism in Arizona made him notorious across America, although only one homicide at his hands can be proved and he insisted 'all I ever did was forced on me and I was tried for and honorably acquitted of' (*Leadville Democrat*, 1884: 1495). In his last years, Holliday eked a living gambling in Colorado mining camps and health resorts. He died of tuberculosis in a spa-town hotel in 1887, only thirty-six years old.

Given that he lived with the disease throughout his adult life, some biomedical knowledge of tuberculosis might illuminate Holliday's experiences. The organism *Mycobacterium tuberculosis* is spread by coughing, and the lungs are the most common site of disease. The course of tuberculosis is typically chronic; as the disease progresses over weeks or months, the patient suffers exhaustion, chest pain, night-sweats, and weight-loss to the point of emaciation. Coughing and breathlessness become increasingly debilitating as cavities and scarring replace healthy lung tissue (Williams and Williams, 1871: 1–11; Davies, 2003: 108–24). Effective antibiotics were not developed until the 1940s: although they could survive several years after diagnosis (Newsholme, 1908: 449–50), late-Victorian consumptives usually died between the ages of fifteen and thirty-five (Dubos and Dubos, 1996: appendix D).

Friends suggested Holliday weighed around forty pounds less than the average late-Victorian man of his height ('Doc Holliday', 1882: 6; Squire, 1893: 189), and described him as 'a slender, sickly fellow' (*Arizona Daily Star*, 1882), 'emaciated and bent' ('Death of J. A. [sic] Holliday', 1887). Travelling to New Mexico in 1878, he became too sick to be moved for ten days (Mary Cummings' statement, 1977: 76); in 1882, he was fit enough to ride around Arizona hunting outlaws but, by 1884, he had recurring pneumonia, weighed only 122 pounds ('Holliday bound over', 1884: 4), and was described as 'weak, out of health, sprits and money, slowly dying' (*Leadville Democrat*, 1884: 1494) – although he survived another three years. Like many American consumptives, he managed his symptoms by drinking heavily (Davis, 1891: 120). His condition was debilitating, life-limiting, and conspicuous enough to influence his social interactions.

Nonetheless, the insight offered by such medical knowledge is limited for two reasons. First, experiences of disability are shaped by socioeconomic and cultural context as much as by biology (Hughes, 2002: 61; Lawlor, 2006: 6–7). In an 1884 interview, Holliday conveyed his frightening physical disadvantage in the violent, competitive saloon subculture, but his complaints focused on his violent associates, not his impairment: in a different setting, physical weakness might have been irrelevant (*Leadville Democrat*, 1884: 1495).

Second, while biomedical narratives would soon dominate attitudes toward disability, oppressing people with impairment by reducing them to pathological objects and naturalising their social marginalisation (Williams, 2001: 125–27; Hughes, 2002: 59), biomedicine did not achieve this absolute power to define and determine consumptive identity during Holliday's lifetime. Even after Robert Koch's 1882 announcement that tuberculosis was contagious, a Colorado newspaper stated that the 'bacillus' was 'inherited' ('Talks', 1886: 4), and another journalist even claimed Holliday was 'slowly dying of a bullet that had pierced his lungs' (*Leadville Democrat*, 1884: 1494). The biomedical model of tuberculosis was still too poorly understood to wholly determine how people responded to consumptives or how consumptives perceived themselves.

Instead, early depictions of Holliday deployed rudimentary, incoherent biomedical concepts as convenient supplements to more established sentimental, religious or Romantic models of consumption. Traditional consumptive stereotypes were ostensibly benign; they assumed a correspondence between physical and emotional traits, and combined an ideal of the Christian 'good death' with more secular Romantic associations between consumption and creativity, sincerity, and sensitivity (Lawlor, 2006: 35–38, 53–58, 114–15). Even medical texts in the 1880s still relied on these archaic ideas to define a 'consumptive type' of person (see Galton and Mahomed, 1882).

Of course, applying familiar consumptive stereotypes to Holliday was difficult given the inconsistency between his delicate appearance and tough character. The *Denver Republican* marvelled that Holliday's appearance was:

> [A]s different as could be from the generally conceived idea of a killer. Holliday is a slender man [...]. His face is thin and his hair sprinkled heavily with gray. His features are well formed and there is nothing remarkable in them save a well-defined look of determination from his eyes, which the veriest amateur in physiognomy could hardly mistake. His hands are small and soft like a woman's, but the work they have done is anything but womanly.
>
> ('Awful Arizona', 1882)

The typical 'killer' (like the typical 'consumptive') is supposed to possess a particular agreement of temperamental and physical traits. Holliday's persona disrupts expectations and sends the *Republican* reporter swerving between contradictions and qualifications. However, journalists could use contemporary biomedical concepts to cut through these inconsistencies and read his impaired body more 'scientifically'. Holliday's friend E.D. Cowen recalled:

> A person unfamiliar with Holliday's deeds and unstudied in physiognomy would pass him by as a specimen of human insignificance, for he was as frail and as harmless a looking being as ever wielded the pestle of a pharmacy mortar or measured calico behind the retail counter.
>
> Holliday was of medium stature and blonde complexion. He was small boned and of that generally slumped appearance common to sufferers from inherited pulmonary disease. The clenched setting of his finely-pointed lower jaw and the steadiness of his blue eyes were the only features really striking of his pallid countenance. He was scrupulously neat and precise in his attire, though neither a lady's man nor a dandy.
>
> (Cowen, 1898: 5)

The fair, vulnerable, Romantic consumptive survives alongside a newer biomedical concept of 'pulmonary disease'. Crucially, both Cowen and the *Republican* turn to the contemporary pseudo-science of physiognomy to make sense of Holliday, dissecting his body to separate the accidental features (like delicate bones, faded hair, and diseased lungs) from significant features supposed to reveal his true identity (i.e., jaw and eyes). With a systematic approach to reading, categorising and describing impaired bodies, the pseudo-science of the 1880s promised some clarity *and validation* for the consumptive gunfighter, rather than dehumanisation or oppression.

Indeed, the only recorded comment that Holliday made about his illness suggests that, rather than being its victim, he could appropriate a biomedical model of disability to defend his life. Having shot a man who threatened to beat him, Holliday told the court:

> I thought my life was as good to me as his was to him. [...] I knew that I would be a child in his hands if he got hold of me; I weigh 122 pounds; I think Allen weighs 170 pounds. I have had the pneumonia three or four times; I don't think I was able to protect myself against him.
>
> ('Holliday bound over', 1884: 4)

For Holliday, the biomedical model's assumption that impairment causes disability was not entirely oppressive: it gave him a precise, credible language with which to explain the consequences of his physical difference in an official setting where his disadvantage might otherwise be ignored. Crucially, he did not regard these biomedical details as incompatible with an assertion that he valued his life.

Nonetheless, contemporary depictions of Holliday are most remarkable for their emphasis on the sick body not pathologised by science but refined through exquisite dress. According to an 1883 description:

[Holliday] was not feeling very well during his temporary sojourn in [Arizona], and, while there was a fertile field for his peculiar talents, the small number of his victims should be attributed to the bad state of health he experienced while there, being a victim of consumption. [...] He is a thin, spare looking man; his iron gray hair is always well combed and oiled; his boots usually wear an immaculate polish; his beautiful scarf, with an elegant diamond pin in the center, looks well on his glossy shirt front, and he prides himself on always keeping scrupulously neat and clean.

('Leadville sketches', 1883)

This account notes Holliday's pathetic status as 'a victim of consumption' and its incompatibility with violence. However, it places more emphasis on the deliberate precision with which he organises his appearance: his meticulous grooming, 'beautiful' costume and carefully placed pin, and his self-conscious pride in neatness and artifice. Here, as in Cowen's account, the phrase *scrupulously neat* is associated with firmness and control.

Although Cowen denied that Holliday was 'a dandy', he may have been equating dandyism with Irish fop Oscar Wilde (1854–1900), who visited Denver one month before Cowen met Holliday there in 1882 (*Rocky Mountain news*, 1882; see George, 2004: 7, on denials of dandyism among exemplary dandies). In fact, these depictions of Holliday recall the restrained, elegant dandyism of Beau Brummell (1778–1840), Max Beerbohm (1872–1954) and, most pertinently, consumptive artist Aubrey Beardsley (1872–1898). Matthew Sturgis suggests that Beardsley used dandyism to assert control over his deteriorating body (Sturgis, 1998: 96–97). It is possible that Holliday's dandyism fulfilled a similar function. In a photograph (Figure 2.1, c.1880), Holliday stands primly, ankles crossed, holding a small book or purse, and seems to be wearing glasses. His dainty pose and close-fitting coat display the thinness of the consumptive body while encasing it in a carapace of regimented buttons: physical frailty is not denied, but it is emphatically *managed*.

The prolonged, intimate process by which Holliday constructed his costume may also be interpreted as a personal and public acceptance – even celebration – of the consumptive body. Contemporaries observed admiringly that '[h]is clothes were custom made' ('Murderer's methods', 1882) – the mark of '[t]he genuine dandy' (Shannon, 2006: 135). His choice of bespoke tailoring means that, rather than hurriedly concealing his sick body under cheap, shapeless clothes, Holliday lavished time and money on being measured, fitted, *and re-fitted* for unique garments expressing his personal taste and sculpted precisely to his body. This is a personal act with no ostensible political intent, and yet it has political significance in publicly transforming the impaired body from an object of sentimental pity (Klages, 1999: 196) or pathological scrutiny to a work of art constructed and displayed by the disabled person himself. Unfortunately, the consumptive's assertion of agency in self-presentation would not be appreciated much longer.

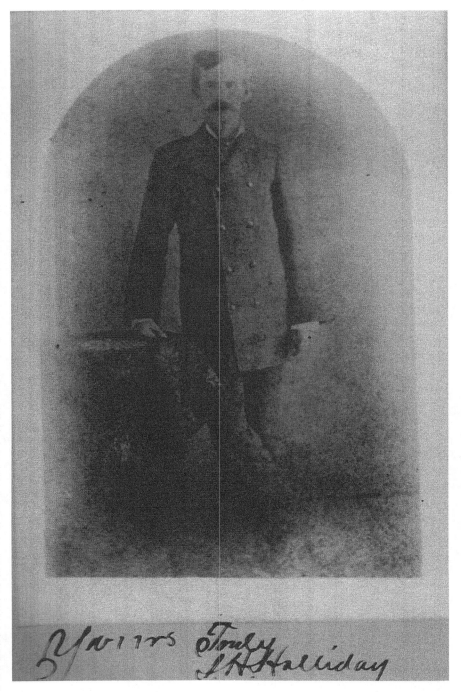

Figure 2.1 Photograph supplied courtesy of the Tombstone Times, Arizona, USA

Decline: twentieth-century tuberculosis

In the 1900s, attitudes toward people with tuberculosis changed dramatically. Thomas J. Mays said 'the position of sufferers from this disease has actually been made unbearable'; they were 'tabooed at hotels, boarding houses and health resorts' and 'frequently the victims of neglect on the part of their friends and families' (Mays, 1905: 1). Driven by (delayed) public panic about contagion, this impairment-specific stigma also coincided with the increasing dominance of a biomedical model of disability that evaluates a person's life by the extent of her or his impairment (Bradock and Parish, 2001: 12). Carol Gill argues that this actively disables people with incurable impairments by 'send[ing] a message that our lives are untenable' (Gill, 2006: 184). Little wonder that Sheila Rothman found that the journals of twentieth-century American TB patients were 'often self-deprecatory and angry [...] suffused with bitterness' (Rothman, 1995: 6) and, by 1955, an English psychiatric survey found that 54 per cent had significant anxiety and depression; they were tormented by their 'uselessness, their unwantedness, their anticipation of rejection' (Wittkower, 1995: 26–27).

In an increasingly hostile climate, representations of Holliday began to project negative attitudes retrospectively. In 1907, his former friend 'Bat' Masterson declared:

> Physically Doc Holliday was a weakling who could not have whipped a healthy fifteen-year-old boy in a go-as-you-please fist fight, and no one knew this better than himself, and the knowledge of this fact was perhaps why he was so ready to resort to a weapon of some kind whenever he got himself into difficulty.
> [...] It was easy to see that he was not a healthy man for he not only looked the part, but he incessantly coughed it as well.
>
> (Masterson, 1907: 35–36, 39–40)

While writers of the 1880s described Holliday's fragility and neatness in loving detail, Masterson gleefully imagines a scenario in which Holliday could be battered. He associates weakness with viciousness, and reference to 'incessant' coughing also implies impatience or distaste not apparent in earlier texts.

Similarly, while writers of the 1880s were surprised that a consumptive would court danger, writers across the twentieth century implied it was inevitable. Stuart Lake's 1931 biography of heroic lawman Wyatt Earp fabricated a quote from Earp concerning Holliday's 'fatalistic courage, a courage induced, I suppose, by the nature of Holliday's disease and the realization that he hadn't long to live, anyway' (Lake, 1994: 196). Paula Mitchell Marks's study of the OK Corral gunfight twice declared that Holliday was suicidal because he 'was dying, anyway' (Marks, 1989: 36, 86). Crucially, neither Lake nor Marks offered real evidence – but, with the notable exception of Roberts (2006), many historians, novelists, and filmmakers followed their lead unquestioningly (Tankard, 2013).

Marks's book preceded two films about Holliday, and Lake worked as a Hollywood consultant (Farager, 1995: 154–61). Their casual dismissal of Holliday's life manifested itself in unusual ways on screen. Six major movie representations of Doc Holliday appeared between 1946 and 1994: Victor Mature in *My Darling Clementine* (1946); Kirk Douglas in *Gunfight at the OK Corral* (1957); Jason Robards in *Hour of the Gun* (1967); Stacy Keach in *Doc* (1971); Val Kilmer in *Tombstone* (1993); and Dennis Quaid in *Wyatt Earp* (1994). During this period, tuberculosis went from being a dreaded incurable disease to a curable disease that seemed close to eradication in the developed world; then, in the 1990s, ominous hints of resurgence were both exacerbated and overshadowed by HIV/AIDS (Dormandy, 1999: 361–75, 384–86) – but despite these upheavals, filmmakers were remarkably consistent in refusing to depict a realistically tubercular body on screen. All six actors cough occasionally, but five look sturdy and strong. David Bowie was an early choice for *Tombstone* (Blake, 2007: 162), reflecting the original screenplay's emphasis on Doc's vulnerability in a violent society (Jarre, 1993: 3), but interest in this theme obviously waned and, like *Clementine* and *Gunfight*, *Tombstone* cast an actor whose physique was the most extreme opposite of Holliday's. The body that featured so prominently in texts before 1900 was resolutely denied – with one significant exception.

'It happened that way'?: the tubercular body in *Wyatt Earp*

Regarding his preparation for *Wyatt Earp*, Quaid explained:

> Victims of tuberculosis have a tendency to be very skinny people, and I'm an actor that... I work from the outside in. And I feel like when I play real people [...] I have to have a total commitment to portraying them and getting as close to them as I can. I was 182 pounds, and I was pretty robust and healthy, and so I had to change my physical appearance, and I wound up losing 43 pounds
> ('It happened that way', 1994)

Quaid's Doc is emaciated, tottering on his feet, coughing and wheezing as if his lungs are liquefying inside. His physique affects his interaction with other actors: at one point, Morgan Earp defuses an argument between Doc and a cowboy by simply lifting Doc and carrying him away, and Doc's enraged, impotent squirming conveys the weaker man's humiliation by the stronger. In fact, on two separate occasions, Holliday did shoot stronger men who manhandled or threatened to beat him ('Holliday bound over', 1884: 4; Roberts, 2006: 128), so Quaid's physical appearance reflects an important aspect of Holliday's motivation as a gunfighter.

Quaid assumed that recreating embodied experience would give the most direct access to the historical Holliday. Yet Lawlor points out that, while the biology of tuberculosis determines the rough parameters of consumptive experience, the details and meanings of that experience are historically-specific (Lawlor, 2006: 6–7). In *Wyatt Earp*, the cultural framework giving meaning to Doc's bodily symptoms is a dehistoricised biomedical model of tuberculosis and of disability. Characters even declare Doc is 'dying of tuberculosis' – a term I have never seen used in descriptions of Holliday during his lifetime.

Far from illuminating life with chronic illness in the 1880s, the spectacle of a vividly, painfully rotting tubercular body is accompanied by dialogue that 'proves' biological impairment causes suffering, and that the lives of those so afflicted are invalid. Quaid's Doc tells Wyatt he welcomes death because 'I know it can't be any worse for me', and 'I'm dead anyway, so if you want to go out in a blaze of glory, I'm with you'. Astonishingly, the film is so adamant that Doc is 'dead anyway' that it stages *and then contradicts* frontier actor Eddie Foy's famous eye-witness account of Holliday diving to the floor to avoid gunfire in Kansas in the 1870s (Roberts, 2006: 97). Marks stated (without citing evidence) that this dive was at odds with Holliday's 'suicidal tendencies' (Marks, 1989: 86). *Wyatt Earp* actually 'corrects' Foy's account in a way that matches Marks's expectations and shows Doc sitting stubbornly in a hail of bullets while everyone else ducks.

In *Wyatt Earp*, Doc is completely disposable: with no goodbye scene between the friends, Doc is simply dropped from the film when Wyatt moves on, and his death is acknowledged only by a piece of floating text at the end stating (inaccurately) that he 'died in a sanitarium'. This is not an insignificant error. Two major biographies available to the filmmakers suggested that Holliday died in a spa-town hotel, not a medical institution (Myers, 1973: 209; Jahns, 1998: 282), but *Wyatt Earp* contradicts this with a twentieth-century ideal of institutional segregation for people with tuberculosis. Although only a minority actually entered institutions, post-1900 American consumptives were redefined as 'TB patients' who required professional medical supervision (Ott, 1996: 136–37), and the TB sanitarium dominated discourses of and attitudes toward tuberculosis to the extent that four of the six films refer to Holliday dying in a sanitarium – as if the truth was simply inconceivable.

Perhaps most troubling is *Wyatt Earp*'s decision to deny Holliday's dandyish poise. Quaid is grimy, uncouth, and shouts crude insults at ladies. The film depicts unforgivable lapses in grooming and hygiene; his coat is stained, he never wears a tie (much less a 'beautiful scarf') and, most pertinently, he coughs (loudly, wetly, spitting) into a filthy rag instead of a white linen handkerchief: he is contagious and unclean. This may be consistent with the film's grimy aesthetic but, far from being 'authentic', the grime directly contradicts eye-witness descriptions of Holliday. It evokes twentieth-century anxieties about contagion in a setting where such anxieties were negligible ('Talks', 1886: 4), and through an individual who was regarded as extraordinarily clean.

Perhaps Holliday's personal style was essentially inconsistent with a biomedical model of tuberculosis or disability – and, for the filmmakers, the biomedical model was powerful enough to override historical evidence. *Wyatt Earp*'s insistence that the incurable tubercular body is unclean and disposable throws into relief Holliday's insistence that the consumptive body (however fragile) is immaculate and precious.

Conclusion

Social attitudes toward tuberculosis and disability have changed almost beyond recognition since Holliday died in 1887. Quaid's well-meaning commitment to presenting a realistically tubercular body on screen reveals how far its meaning differs from that of the nineteenth-century consumptive. There is no reason to suspect that the convulsive coughing, spitting, and extreme emaciation exhibited by Quaid were not features of Holliday's illness, but his acquaintances in the 1880s perceived the same symptoms in a different cultural framework.

Holliday's friends did describe his condition (physical, emotional, and social) in 1884 in pitying terms. More often, though, their impressions were dominated by his genteel manners and exquisite dress and grooming. At the end of his life, fourteen years of tuberculosis, substance abuse, and a precarious existence among violent frontier gamblers had left him 'emaciated and bent', and prematurely grey – and yet two separate articles still described him as 'rather good looking' ('Doc Holliday', 1886; 'Death of a notorious bunco man', 1887). The body *Wyatt Earp* presents as loathsome and disposable was once seen as 'delicate', 'scrupulously neat', and appealing.

To convey Holliday's unique disabled identity to a modern audience, future filmmakers should not embrace a biomedical model of disability uncritically. Biomedical discourses are not universal, timeless or objective; rather, in presenting themselves as such, they marginalise and invalidate more appropriate perspectives. While exploring the impact of disability on Holliday's experiences is quite necessary, filmmakers should be aware that a modern audience's interpretation of tubercular symptoms will probably be informed by medical discoveries and social stigma that emerged after Holliday's death. It would be absurd to deny Holliday's impairment – to cast another burly action hero – but an emaciated, coughing consumptive body must be placed in a context informed by historically appropriate sentimentality and Romanticism, not by modern medical anxieties.

Early descriptions of Holliday tell us little about his medical condition, but a great deal about how his physical presence was experienced by his friends. Above all, Holliday's contemporaries appreciated his determination to design and present himself *just so*. It is this meticulous, scrupulous agency, more than any tubercular symptom, which captures the disruptive potential of Holliday's identity as the suave disabled gunfighter.

References

Arizona Daily Star (1882), 30 May [transcription online] Available www. tombstonehistoryarchives.com/?page_id=14 (accessed 29 July 2011).

Awful Arizona (1882) *Denver Republican*, 22 May.

Baur, J. (1959) The health seeker in the Westward movement, 1830–1900, *Mississippi Valley Historical Review*, 91–110.

Blake, M. (2007) *Hollywood and the OK Corral*, Jefferson: McFarland.

Bradock, D. and Parish, S. (2001) An institutional history of disability, in G. Albrecht, K. Seelman, and M. Bury (eds) *Handbook of Disability Studies*, Thousand Oaks: Sage.

Caught in Denver (1882) *Denver Republican*, 16 May.

Courtwright, D. (1996) *Violent Land: Single Men and Social Disorder from the Frontier to the Inner City*, Cambridge: Harvard University Press.

Cowen, E.D. (1898) Happy bad men of the west: a reminiscence, *Salt Lake Herald*, 14 November, 5.

Davies, P. (2003) Respiratory tuberculosis, in P. Davies, *Clinical Tuberculosis*, London: Arnold.

Davis, N. (1891) *Consumption: How to Prevent it and How to Live with it*, Philadelphia: F.A. Davis.

Death of a notorious bunco man (1887) *New York Sun*, November 20.

Death of J.A. [sic] Holliday (1887), in B.T. Traywick (1996) *John Henry: the 'Doc' Holliday story*, Tombstone: Red Marie's bookstore.

Doc Holliday (1882) *Atlanta Weekly Constitution*, 27 June, p. 6.

Doc Holliday (1886) *St Joseph Herald*, July 16.

Dormandy, T. (1999) *The White Death: A History of Tuberculosis*, London: Hambledon and London.

Dubos, R. and Dubos, J. (1996) *The White Plague: Tuberculosis, Man and Society*, New Brunswick: Rutgers University Press.

Farager, J. (1995) The tale of Wyatt Earp: seven films, in T. Mico, J. Miller-Monzon, and D. Rubel (eds) *Past Imperfect: History According to the Movies*, London: Cassel.

Galton, F. and Mahomed, F.A. (1882) An inquiry into the physiognomy of phthisis by the method of 'composite portraiture', *Guys Hospital Reports*, 25, 475–93.

George, L. (2004) The emergence of the dandy, *Literature Compass*, 1, 1–13.

Gill, C. (2006) Disability, constructed vulnerability, and socially constructed palliative care, *Journal of Palliative Care*, 22, Autumn, 183–91.

Holliday bound over (1884) *Leadville Daily Herald*, 26 August, p. 4.

Hughes, B. (2002) Disability and the body, in C. Barnes, M. Oliver, and L. Barton (eds) *Disability Studies Today*, Cambridge: Polity Press.

It happened that way (1994) in *Wyatt Earp*, dir. by Lawrence Kasdan, Warner/Tig/Kasdan [2004 DVD].

Jahns, P. (1998) *The Frontier World of Doc Holliday* [1957], Lincoln, London: University of Nebraska Press.

Jarre, K. (1993) *Tombstone: An Original Screenplay*, fourth draft, March 15. Online, available: www.dailyscript.com/scripts/tombstone.pdf (accessed December 22, 2011).

Klages, M. (1999) *Woeful Afflictions: Disability and Sentimentality in Victorian America*, Philadelphia: University of Pennsylvania Press.

Lake, S. (1994) *Wyatt Earp: Frontier Marshal* [1931], New York: Pocket.

Lawlor, C. (2006) *Consumption and Literature: The Making of the Romantic Disease*, Basingstoke: Palgrave Macmillan.

Leadville Democrat [August 20, 1884], in D. Griswold and J. Griswold, (1996), *History of Leadville and Lake County, Colorado*, Boulder: Colorado Historical Society/ University of Colorado Press, 1494–95.

Leadville sketches by a former resident, *Omaha Daily Bee*, (10 May, 1883), 2.

Marks, P.M. (1989) *And Die in the West: The Story of the OK Corral Gunfight*, New York: Simon and Schuster.

Mary Cummings's statement: the OK Corral fight at Tombstone: a footnote by Kate Elder, (1977) Bork, A.W. and Boyer, G. (eds) *Arizona and the West*, 19.

Mays, T.J. (1905) *The Fly and Tuberculosis*, New York: A. R. Elliot.

Murderer's methods (1882) *Denver Daily Tribune*, 16 May.

Myers, J. (1973), *Doc Holliday* [London: 1957], Lincoln: University of Nebraska Press.

Newsholme, A. (1908) *The Prevention of Tuberculosis*, London: Methuen.

Ott, K. (1996) *Fevered Lives: Tuberculosis and American Culture since 1870*, Cambridge: Harvard University Press.

Roberts, G. (2006) *Doc Holliday: The Life and Legend*, Hoboken: Wiley and Sons.

Rocky Mountain News (1882), 16 April.

Rothman, S. (1995) *Living in the Shadow of Death: Tuberculosis and the Social Experience of Illness in American History*, Baltimore: John Hopkins University Press.

Shannon, B. (2006) *The Cut of his Coat: Men, Dress and Consumer Culture in Britain, 1860–1914*, Athens: Ohio University Press.

Squire, J. (1893) *The Hygienic Prevention of Consumption*, London: Charles Griffin.

Sturgis, M. (1998) *Aubrey Beardsley: A Biography*, London: Harper Collins.

Talks about tubercles (1886) *Buena Vista Democrat*, 19 May, p. 4.

Tankard, A. (2013) 'He laughed at death, while courting its embrace': reconstructing Doc Holliday's experience of illness, *WWHA*, VI, 4, 3–14.

Williams, C.J.B. and Williams, C.T. (1871) *Pulmonary Consumption*, London: Longmans, Green and Co.

Williams, G. (2001) Theorizing disability, in L. Gary, G. Albrecht, K. Seelman, and M. Bury (eds) *Handbook of Disability Studies*, Thousand Oaks: Sage.

Wittkower, E. (1995) *A Psychiatrist Looks at Tuberculosis*, London: NAPT.

Wyatt Earp (1994), dir. by Lawrence Kasdan, Warner/Tig/Kasdan [2004 DVD].

3 'Beings in another galaxy'

Historians, the Nazi 'euthanasia' programme, and the question of opposition

Emmeline Burdett

The phrase *beings in another galaxy* was used by the historian Richard Grunberger in *A Social History of the Third Reich* (1971). He used the phrase to explain why the Nazi persecution of the Jews – unlike the so-called euthanasia programme – attracted no official protests. He argued that while the victims of Nazi euthanasia were representatives of every part of society, there was a widespread perception among Germans that Jewish suffering affected beings that were utterly separate from themselves. This chapter shows that a parallel perception was – and in some respects still is – in operation among Anglo-American historians of the Nazi period. It is my contention that, for some decades, the most enduring response to the programme has been to emphasise the protests against it, to the complete exclusion of both the programme and its victims.

At the Nuremberg Medical Trial, the euthanasia programme was described as the 'systematic and secret execution of the aged, insane, incurably ill, of deformed children and other persons, by gas, lethal injection and diverse other means, in nursing homes, hospitals and asylums' (NMT Indictment, 1946–1947: Paragraph 9, FO 646). The indictment estimated that the perpetrators of the Nazi euthanasia programme had murdered hundreds of thousands of people. The ideas underpinning this non-consensual killing of those perceived to be an unproductive drain on society's resources can be traced back through the wider Western history of eugenics, as well as the Nazis' systematic devaluation of disabled people. Indeed, prior to the beginning of the euthanasia programme, this devaluation expressed itself in many ways: the 1933 Law for the Prevention of Congenitally Diseased Offspring – enforced sterilisation, portrayed as a 'voluntary sacrifice' made by those born 'defective'; mathematics questions in school textbooks portraying disabled lives in terms of crude 'cost-benefit analysis'; and propaganda films ranging from the insidious *Ich Klage an (I Accuse)* to sensationalist documentaries shot in institutions, openly disputing the humanity of the inmates (Burleigh, 1994: 183–219).

The programme itself began in 1938 with a request to Hitler from the father of the 'Knauer baby' – an infant who, it was claimed, was blind, missing a part of one leg and one arm, and was, allegedly, an 'idiot' (Burleigh, 1994: 98–99). A backdated authorisation for so-called mercy-killing was issued soon after the outbreak of the Second World War, and the killing of children and adults began in earnest. There were six killing centres – Bernburg, Brandenburg, Grafeneck, Hadamar, Hartheim, and Sonnenstein. These closed after Church-led protests in 1941, but decentralised 'wild euthanasia' continued until 1945 (Friedlander, 1995: 151). This last point is vital, as I now show that for decades, study of the Nazi euthanasia programme has been hindered – if not totally prevented – by historians' casual dismissal of the murder of some hundreds of thousands of people by their exclusive focus on the protests against the programme, which supposedly brought it to an end.

'Outraged human feelings': from 1950 to 1970

It has been claimed that, in the decades immediately following the end of World War II, German historians paid no meaningful attention to the Nazi euthanasia programme, the only one dealing with it being Alice Platen Hallermund (Burleigh, 1991: 318). Reading between the lines of Burleigh's article, however, gives rise to the suspicion that, in the early years at least, the Nazi euthanasia programme was not regarded as being a subject of great interest and importance by many *non*-German historians either. A number of explanations have been put forward to suggest why this situation might have arisen, such as a combination of the euthanasia programme simply having been overlooked due to the sheer volume of atrocities committed by the Nazis, and the tendency of historians to pay more attention to crimes committed against Jews and people of occupied nations than against German civilians (Mühlberger, 1997: 553).

By contrast, doubts have been cited among historians and the public as to the criminal nature of killing people who are frequently perceived to be a burden on society, as opposed to active participants and contributors (Kudlick, 2003). This chapter builds on Kudlick's explanation and argues that historians have perceived the victims of the Nazi euthanasia programme in ways that are commensurate with the ways in which disabled people are perceived in their societies. For example, during the decades in which disabled people were in the main confined to homes or long-stay hospitals, with little opportunity to integrate with an inaccessible society, historians have tended to perceive the Nazi euthanasia programme as a dry ethical issue, not a programme of systematic murder. Consequently, it makes a kind of sense that these historians should either ignore the programme altogether or emphasise the protests to it, as though the victims themselves were not real. The writer and disability rights activist Jenny Morris explored Miller and Gwynne's 1972 comment that institutionalisation was 'social death', and this comment is taken to a whole new level when it is considered in conjunction with historians' dismissive attitudes to the murder of tens of thousands of people (Morris, 1993: 130–31).

Early works on Nazism (Trevor-Roper, 1953; Bullock, 1964; Shirer, 1964) make no reference at all to the euthanasia programme. Shirer does include an extensive section on the Nuremberg Medical Trial, but this appears in a section of the book dealing with Nazi medical experiments, and makes no mention of the euthanasia programme.

A quite different approach is taken by historians of the same period, whose focus is not on Nazi Germany in general, but on the Nazi persecution of the Jews. These historians highlight the Catholic Church-led protests against the euthanasia programme that supposedly (although not in fact) brought it to an end. In addition, they advance the view – expressed by Grunberger at the beginning of this chapter – that the euthanasia programme was primarily an example of the resistance that Germans could mount to Nazi policies if they felt that the victims thereof were sufficiently similar to themselves to be worthy of protection. Reitlinger writes that 'an *asocial* person, although a nuisance, might still be a German. If, however, that asocial belonged to a subject race, public opinion was dumb' (Reitlinger, 1953: 126). Leon Poliakov ploughs a very similar furrow:

> Here again we must understand what is meant by 'human feelings'. The instructive example of the 'euthanasia program' indicates clearly enough how the 'will of the people', German public opinion, was able to be an active and effective factor … We have seen how … this other extermination programme … had to be stopped because of the outcry against it of a population whose 'human feelings' it had outraged. Also, the extermination of the so-called 'useless mouths' concerned German lives that were flesh of their flesh.
>
> (Poliakov, 1956: 282–83)

Strikingly similar sentiments are to be found in Guenther Lewy's *The Catholic Church and Nazi Germany* (1964):

> But the large majority of the very people who had been outraged when their sons and daughters, brothers and sisters, had been put to death, failed to react in the same manner when their Jewish neighbours were deported and eventually killed in the very gas chambers designed for and first tried out in the euthanasia program … That German public opinion and the Church were a force to be reckoned with in principle and could have played a role in the Jewish disaster as well is the principle lesson to be derived from the fate of Hitler's euthanasia program.
>
> (Lewy, 1964: 265–67)

Reitlinger, Poliakov, and Lewy make the common claim that, because of their anti-Semitism, the German public and the Catholic Church in Germany did not defend Jews who were being systematically persecuted by the Nazis. They make the further claim that, as the example of the protests against the Nazi euthanasia programme shows, protests on behalf of persecuted Jews would, quite possibly, have been sufficient to halt the Final Solution in its tracks.

There are, however, a number of unspoken assumptions underlying the claims, and it is important to investigate these before proceeding. Poliakov and Lewy in particular emphasise the close relationships between victims of the Nazi euthanasia programme, and those who protested against it. Furthermore, their words make it appear that the euthanasia victims' position in society had always previously been a very secure one. This ignores the whole history of eugenic thought in Europe and the United States, which originated with Francis Galton and gathered momentum in response to such things as the carnage of World War I.

Uncovering the history of eugenics has been an endeavour carried out by much later historians, but the three to which I refer had an awareness of it. For example, Lewy makes a comparison between the Nazis' Law for the Prevention of Hereditarily Diseased Offspring, passed in 1933, and the contemporaneous sterilisation laws that were in operation in various American states:

> During the first year of the Law's operation [the Law for the Prevention of Hereditarily Diseased Offspring] 32,268 sterilizations were carried out; in 1935, 73,714 persons were sterilized, and 63,547 in 1936. Each of these last figures was higher than the number sterilized in over fifty years in the United States, where from the enactment of the first sterilization law in 1907 until 1958, 60,166 sterilizations took place; furthermore, some of these were voluntary.
>
> (Lewy, 1964: 265–67)

This statement raises a number of questions – not least, how voluntary is a choice to have oneself sterilised if one lives in a society in which sterilisation is promoted as desirable for certain types of people? Nevertheless, Lewy's argument attempts to close off questions about eugenics in the United States, and eugenics in general.

Lewy, Poliakov, and Reitlinger have all argued that the refusal of non-Jewish Germans to speak out on behalf of persecuted Jews, while protesting vehemently about the euthanasia programme, can be explained by pointing to the anti-Semitism of those same non-Jewish Germans. The leap that none of the three historians make is to question whether the precarious position of Jews as Other was in any way replicated in the case of groups subjected to sterilisation. Lewy's comments about sterilisation, as well as the three historians' claims about the victims of the euthanasia programme being 'flesh of their flesh' in relation to non-Jewish Germans, makes it appear that neither the American nor German sterilisation policies were accompanied by any sort of promotion or propaganda that may have contributed to a climate in which those targeted by the policies were systematically devalued. This is essentially a question about whether measures aimed at eradicating impairment constitute prejudice. As I now demonstrate, the question is an enduring one.

A continuing trend: from 1970 to 1990

Like William Shirer's *The Rise and Fall of the Third Reich*, Grunberger's *A Social History of the Third Reich* appears to have met with popular rather than scholarly success. Grunberger's book is divided into sections, each of which discusses an aspect of daily life under the Nazi regime (e.g., 'Cinema' and 'Health'). Grunberger discusses the Nazi euthanasia programme at length, and it quickly becomes clear that, in his view, its importance lies in the German public's reaction to it (portrayed as one of universal condemnation) rather than in the fact that the programme was implemented and resulted in the murder of at least tens of thousands of people. Grunberger also refers persistently to the programme as 'mercy-killing'. This take on the programme's importance is evident from the very first time Grunberger mentions it:

> The realization of what war and occupation meant to the occupied dawned only on a few Germans, and – unlike the euthanasia killings of German incurables and mental defectives – never agitated public opinion.
>
> (Grunberger, 1971: 52)

Here, we can see that Grunberger is making use of the arguments first employed by Reitlinger, Lewy, and Poliakov, in order to show that the only noteworthy aspect of the Nazi euthanasia programme is the protests against it, which were by implication universal. However, after stopping briefly to describe the euthanasia programme as the 'wartime mercy-killing of the mentally and physically handicapped' (Grunberger, 1971: 283), Grunberger reveals two pieces of information, both of which call into question the implied universality of the protests against it:

> *Ich Klage an* ('I Accuse') was a Nazi propaganda film which told the fictional story of a young woman who, after being diagnosed with multiple sclerosis, implores her physician husband to kill her – a request to which he eventually acquiesces.
>
> (Gallagher, 1990: 92)

Grunberger tells us that the Nazi authorities took note of audience reactions to this film, and he quotes one comment:

> Quite interesting, but in this film the same thing happens as in the asylums where they are finishing off all the lunatics right now. What guarantee have we got that no abuses creep in?
>
> (cited in Grunberger, 1971: 486)

Grunberger describes this comment as 'Delphic', and remarks that what he calls 'this sort of boomerang effect' can also be seen in public reactions to other films:

> The SD reported apprehensions in the ethnically-mixed Eastern provinces that Polish viewers of colonial liberation epics … might be stimulated into identifying themselves with the rebels on the screen.
>
> (Grunberger, 1971: 486)

It is rather difficult to gauge from this what sort of picture Grunberger wants to paint of public reactions to the Nazi euthanasia programme; clearly, what links the comments in the SD reports is a fear that life might begin to imitate art. However, this explanation is unsatisfactory as far as *Ich Klage an* is concerned, as the audience-member interviewed claims that the sort of killing the film portrays is *the same* as that taking place in asylums, thus her or his fear that abuses might occur would seem to relate only to some possible *extension* of these killings. Of course, we do not know what sort of extension the interviewee might have envisaged, and that is possibly why Grunberger describes the comment as 'Delphic'. In any event, unless the SD had managed to uncover the only audience-member at any screening of *Ich Klage an* who was not passionately opposed to what was happening 'in the asylums, where they are finishing off all the lunatics', it would seem that this report, so diligently quoted by Grunberger, provides further evidence that at least one member of the German public must have believed that 'finishing off all the lunatics' did not constitute an 'abuse' of 'euthanasia. Grunberger, however, makes no mention of this interpretation.

The problem of interpretation once more rears its head when Grunberger describes some of the events leading up to the implementation of the Nazi euthanasia programme:

> [I]n preparation for the euthanasia programme the Nazi authorities summoned leading members of university medical faculties to secret recording sessions for *Assessoren*, i.e. selectors of feeble-minded and incurably ill inmates of institutions for mercy-killing. At one such session a medical luminary (Professor Ewald) walked out in protest – but none of his eight fellow-professors followed suit.
>
> (Grunberger, 1971: 397)

This passage is especially important. In common with the other historians mentioned, Grunberger has made clear that its importance lies in the large part played by the German public in its supposed demise. His interest in German attitudes toward Nazi policies having been clearly established, we might expect that Grunberger would have offered some additional discussion of the apparent acceptance of the programme by Professor Ewald's eight colleagues. This is not, however, an avenue that Grunberger sees fit to explore and the discussion of the programme also contains another uncritical use of the phrase *mercy-killing*.

Grunberger's final comment about the Nazi euthanasia programme contains the 'beings in another galaxy' statement to which I refer in the title of this chapter, and he again goes back to his original assessment of how it is not the programme itself that is important, but what the protests against it reveal about German society:

> The feasibility of protests of this nature was demonstrated ... by Cardinal Galen's denunciation of euthanasia from the pulpit ... But the euthanasia victims were flesh of German flesh, and those affected by their deaths ranged through all classes of society ... as far as the great majority were concerned, Jewish suffering affected beings in another galaxy rather than inhabitants of the same planet as themselves.
>
> (Grunberger, 1971: 584–85)

In common with other historians, Grunberger is keen to attribute the German public's failure to protest on behalf of persecuted Jews as an example of that same public's deep-rooted anti-Semitism, but fails to interrogate evidence that calls his view of the universal, monolithic public opposition to the euthanasia programme into question.

Such a view was not only exhibited by popular historians such as Grunberger, but can also be found in more scholarly works such as Ian Kershaw's *Popular Opinion and Political Dissent* (2002). Kershaw's book tells a by now familiar story, in which liberal use is made of the protests against the Nazi euthanasia programme, with the consequence that its victims, its post-1941 continuation, and its moral implications, are totally ignored. We are told that the 'euthanasia action' was set in motion by a secret written order by Hitler shortly after the beginning of the war. By the time the action was officially halted almost two years later, it had claimed the lives of more than 70,000 people. Interspersed with Kershaw's examples of opposition to the Nazi euthanasia programme are brief references to the people who were actually killed (Kershaw, 2002: 338). Nevertheless, this is overwhelmingly a tale of German resistance. The few lines describing the programme itself, set against the twelve-page tale of the resistance to it, render the victims of Nazi euthanasia effectively invisible and irrelevant. It is hardly surprising that Kershaw should conclude that the 'Churches came, in 1941, to lead a victory without parallel in halting the 'euthanasia action' (Kershaw, 2002: 272). Kershaw reveals in a footnote that the programme did not end, but it is hard to envisage that this admission would have had much impact upon the reader. It is also important to note Kershaw's complete failure to mention the propaganda against 'useless eaters', and his lack of discussion of any possible motives for the instigation of Nazi euthanasia. It is as though this programme of systematic murder came, in Kershaw's view, from nowhere, and could be discarded the moment opposition to it began to be heard. This may be partially explicable insofar as the book is largely devoted to a discussion of popular opposition to Nazi policies. Nevertheless, this approach remains another case of the Nazi euthanasia programme being effectively ignored due to historians' desire to focus on opposition, and to regard it as a symbol of the possibility of German resistance to the Nazis, as well as a demonstration of German anti-Semitism.

While Anglo-American historians' studies of different aspects of Nazism widened considerably throughout this period, the attention that these historians devoted to the euthanasia programme remained depressingly unchanged. The idea that it was noteworthy only for the protests against it, which supposedly brought it to an end, was so ingrained that even when, as in the cases of Grunberger and Kershaw, historians were in possession of sources which might reasonably have led them to interrogate their assumptions, this did not happen. Toward the end of this period, studies involving the discussion of Nazi 'medical crimes' began to appear. Of particular note are the books dealing with the broad topic of 'the Nazi doctors', which mentioned the euthanasia programme as part of their wider enquiries into the links between medicine and racism in Nazi Germany. The West German historian Götz Aly is credited with demonstrating that the

Nazi euthanasia programme was not unpopular as, apart from anything else, many parents of impaired children were keen to rid themselves of the stigma that they felt that this entailed (Proctor, 1989: 194). Euthanasia is described as 'an extreme form of racial hygiene' in the sense that its application widened to encompass not 'just' the sick and disabled, but also those from racial groups considered 'inferior' (Weindling, 1989: 9–10). Though Weindling and Proctor are not investigating the programme for itself (Kudlick, 2003: 787, footnote 81), it is noteworthy that both men discuss the programme in terms of a desire to clarify the Nazis racial views, and make no attempt to trivialise it by focusing on the protests against it.

'A bleak subject': from 1990 to the present

In a 1995 edition of the historical journal *Isis*, the English historian Michael Burleigh's book *Death and Deliverance: Euthanasia in Germany 1900–1945* (1994) was described as the 'first full-length examination of what its author rightly terms "a bleak subject"' (Weiss, 1995: 680). This is distinctly odd, as Hugh Gregory Gallagher's book on the same 'bleak' subject – *By Trust Betrayed: Patients, Physicians, and the License to Kill in the Third Reich* – had been published five years earlier. Gallagher's book does not appear in Burleigh's list of secondary sources, and, like Robert Jay Lifton's *The Nazi Doctors*, Shirer's *Rise and Fall of the Third Reich*, and Grunberger's *A Social History of the Third Reich*, seems to have met with public rather than scholarly success. Possible explanations for this discrepancy are Gallagher's use of a team of translators to assist him with his source material, and also that Gallagher eschews the traditional 'objectivity' of the historian and, as it were, writes himself into the story he tells. He tells us that he is a wheelchair-user, as a result of an attack of polio when he was nineteen, and lets us know what he thinks about the relationship between disabled people and the rest of society. His book includes as an afterword his conversation with three young German disability rights activists about the progress of disability rights in Germany and the legacy of Nazism (Gallagher, 1990: 1, 275–81). As *By Trust Betrayed* also contains a chapter discussing 'The Handicapped in Other Times and Places' (Gallagher, 1990: 24–44), it is probably fair to say that it was written with clear socio-political aims in mind.

Gallagher's approach is particularly pertinent to the exploration of changing attitudes toward disability. *By Trust Betrayed* opens with an introduction in which, as well as giving an overview of the book's contents, he writes about the fear he had of impaired people before becoming impaired himself, and about his perceptions of how others see him. In this way, he does exactly the opposite of what the historians seen so far have done. By writing himself into the story he makes it possible for the reader to view the Nazi euthanasia programme *from the point of view of the victims.* This is, as the present chapter shows, something that was simply impossible before. This does not mean that Gallagher obscures the victims – as an obsessive focus on the protests does – but that the reader embarks upon a reading of the book in a certain frame of mind, ready and willing to exercise her or his empathy toward the victims of the euthanasia programme. In addition, Gallagher writes that:

> [A] society's discrimination and cruelty toward the disabled [is] such an intriguing business. The perpetrators are victimizing not some alien religious or ethnic group, but rather their fellow citizens, their own friends and family members, and in due course, themselves.
>
> (Gallagher, 1990: 3)

Furthermore, he writes, 'I have become convinced that the place of the disabled in society needs study. Anthropologists, sociologists, and historians need to investigate the origins and the development of social attitudes and behaviour towards the disabled' (Gallagher, 1990: 3). These statements directly challenge earlier historians' claims and insinuations that the euthanasia programme came from nowhere and that there could obviously be no possibility of the German public demonstrating anything less than one hundred per cent support for those targeted, people who of course reminded them of themselves. Gallagher's chapter 'The Origins of Aktion T4' expands on this, tracing these origins back to the mid-nineteenth century and the 1859 publication of Charles Darwin's work The *Origin of Species*. Gallagher argues that the simplicity of Darwin's theory meant that it could easily be misconstrued. It was, and Darwin's theories were applied to human beings – something Darwin himself did not shrink from (Gallagher, 1990: 76–77).

From the point of view of his discussion of the Nazi euthanasia programme and its origins, Gallagher's book, like Burleigh's and Friedlander's, is a 'full-length study'. The difference among the three books lies principally in the degree of importance they attach to different explanations for the programme. Like *By Trust Betrayed*, Burleigh's *Death and Deliverance: Euthanasia in Germany 1900–1945* (1994) and Henry Friedlander's *The Origins of Nazi Genocide: From Euthanasia to the Final Solution* explicitly link the Nazi euthanasia programme with the wider Western development of eugenics. Unlike Gallagher, both Burleigh and Friedlander write straightforward, evidence-based accounts. Nevertheless, Friedlander's approach is significantly more radical than Burleigh's. For example, Burleigh attaches no importance to the question of the basis of the victims' presence in institutions: 'Such studies of patients as do exist tend to use computers to tot up the proportions of epileptics to schizophrenics among the murdered, an approach I find depressing and worrying' (Burleigh, 1994: 285–86). By contrast, Friedlander appreciates the importance of recognising that the perpetrators may have had self-serving reasons for describing their victims in a particular way:

> As I read through the evidence, I realized that the traditional description of the victims of euthanasia as 'mental patients' [*Geisteskranke*] was inaccurate … Although the victims were institutionalized in state hospitals and nursing homes, only some suffered from mental illness. Many were hospitalized only because they were retarded, blind, deaf, or epileptic, or because they had a

physical deformity. They were handicapped patients, persons who in the United States today are covered by the Act for Disabled Americans.

(Friedlander, 1995: xi)

Taken together, these two statements reveal that in Burleigh's view, there can be no justification for taking account of the medical conditions of people murdered in the Nazi euthanasia programme, as what is required is to understand that the programme entailed the mass-murder of vulnerable people. For Friedlander, by contrast, the victims' medical conditions are important, as their murderers may have altered them for their own ends – although Friedlander does not speculate on what these ends might be.

Conclusion

An indicator of changes in attitudes that these books brought about can be found in what followed them. Extracts from Burleigh's *Death and Deliverance* and/or Friedlander's *The Origins of Nazi Genocide* have appeared in such books as *The Final Solution: Origins and Implementations*, edited by David Cesarani; *The Holocaust: Origins, Implementations, Aftermath*, edited by Omer Bartov; and *Social Outsiders in Nazi Germany*, edited by Robert Gellately and Nathan Stolzfus. It is perhaps this last volume that gives the clearest picture of how far historians' views of the Nazi euthanasia programme have improved, thanks to the work of historians who have finally begun to investigate the programme, rather than simply dismissing it. In Gellately and Stolzfus' editorial introduction, they write:

> When the public got wind of what was happening there was some unrest, but no open protest. Some, but not all, local residents near the killing sites were appalled. One woman wrote to the hospital where her two siblings reportedly died within a few days of each other. She said she accepted the Third Reich, and 'hoped to find peace again' if doctors could assure her that her siblings had been killed by virtue of some law that made it possible to relieve people from their chronic suffering.
>
> (Gellately and Stolzfus, 2001: 11)

But if Burleigh and Friedlander have yielded positive results regarding historians' thinking about the Nazi euthanasia programme, what about Gallagher? When, in 2003, the disability historian Catherine J. Kudlick wrote an article in *The American Historical Review*, she did not refer to Gallagher's book at all, despite the similarity of her argument to the one made over a decade earlier. By contrast, Suzanne E. Evans's *Hitler's Forgotten Victims: The Holocaust and the Disabled* (2007) cites Gallagher quite extensively, in a book written because:

> Remembrance of the mass-slaughter of people with disabilities during the Holocaust is … crucial to an understanding of both (1) how and why people

with disabilities continue to be marginalized in contemporary society and (2) the attitudes and moral failures that allowed the Holocaust to happen.

(Evans, 2007: 20)

The question of the contemporary relevance of the Nazi euthanasia programme is a difficult one. In sharp contrast to Evans's view, in 2001, Gallagher published an article in the *Journal of Disability Policy Studies*. The article, entitled 'What the Nazi "Euthanasia Program" Can Tell Us About Disability Oppression', concluded that:

> [W]e Americans with disabilities have the tools we need to protect and preserve our rights and our liberty. Our oppressed brothers and sisters in Nazi Germany were killed because they had no such tools: *they* were oppressed. We Americans with disabilities will never be oppressed so long as the U.S. constitution exists and we ensure that our rights are enforced.

(Gallagher, 2001: 99)

These questions have not yet gone away and vigilance is still required. But what is clear in this chapter is that the study of the Nazi euthanasia programme has come a tremendously long way, and in doing so, it has mirrored positive changes in social attitudes toward disability.

References

Bullock, A. (1964) *Hitler: A Study in Tyranny*, London: Penguin.

Burleigh, M. (1991) Surveys of developments in the social history of medicine: III euthanasia in the Third Reich: some recent literature, *Social History of Medicine*, 317–27.

Burleigh, M. (1994) *Death and Deliverance: Euthanasia in Germany 1900–1945*, Cambridge: Cambridge University Press.

Evans, S.E. (2007) *Hitler's Forgotten Victims: The Holocaust and the Disabled*, Stroud: Tempus Publishing Ltd.

Friedlander, H. (1995) *The Origins of Nazi Genocide: From Euthanasia to the Final Solution*, Chapel Hill: University of North Carolina Press.

Gallagher, H.G. (1990) *By Trust Betrayed: Patients, Physicians and the License to Kill in the Third Reich*, New York: Henry Holt and Company.

Gallagher, H.G. (2001) What the Nazi 'euthanasia program' can tell us about disability oppression, *Journal of Disability Policy Studies*, 12, 2, 96–99.

Gellately, R. and Stolzfus, N. (eds) (2001) *Social Outsiders in Nazi Germany*, Princeton: Princeton University Press.

Grunberger, R. (1971) *A Social History of the Third Reich*, London: Weidenfeld and Nicolson.

Kershaw, I. (2002) *Popular Opinion and Political Dissent*, Oxford: Oxford University Press.

Kudlick, C.J. (2003) disability history: why we need another 'Other', *American Historical Review*, 108, 3, 763–93.

Lewy, G. (1964) *The Catholic Church and Nazi Germany*, New York: McGraw-Hill Book Company.

Morris, J. (1993) *Pride against Prejudice: Transforming Attitudes to Disability*, London: The Women's Press.

Mühlberger, D. (1997) Review of Michael Burleigh's death and deliverance: euthanasia in Germany 1900–1945, *English Historical Review*, 112, 446, 553–54.

Nuremberg Medical Trial Indictment (1946–1947) *U.S. v Karl Brandt et al.*, F.O. 646 Case 1 Medical, 10–11.

Poliakov, L. (1956) *Harvest of Hate*, London: Erek.

Proctor, R. (1989) *Racial Hygiene: Medicine under the Nazis*, Harvard: Harvard University Press.

Reitlinger, G. (1953) *The Final Solution*, London: Vallentine Mitchell and Co.

Shirer, W. (1964) *The Rise and Fall of the Third Reich*, London: Pan.

Trevor-Roper, H. (1953) *Hitler's Table-talk*, London: Weidenfeld and Nicolson.

Weindling, P. (1989) *Health, Race and German Politics between National Unification and Nazism 1870–1945*, Cambridge: Cambridge University Press.

Weiss, S.F. (1995) Review of Michael Burleigh's death and deliverance: euthanasia in Germany 1900–1945, *Isis*, 86, 4, 680–81.

4   Disability and photojournalism in the age of the image

Alice Hall

Cultural critics have, in recent years, declared that 'ours is the era of the image' or an age of the visual (Louvel, 2008: 31; Siebers, 2010: 121). Taking this widely acknowledged primacy of the visual in popular culture as a starting point, this chapter explores representations of disability in contemporary photojournalism. In particular, it examines the work and media representations of Giles Duley and João Silva to argue that they are producing a new kind of disability portraiture that challenges conventional sensationalist and static visual representations of people with disabilities. Drawing on disability studies and photography theory, I suggest that Duley's and Silva's 'eloquent images' (Hocks and Kendrick, 2005: 1) challenge traditional binaries by creating a dynamic interplay between words and images, and between art and activism.

I argue that Duley and Silva are important figures for thinking about ways in which stories of disability are documented in contemporary journalism and the potential for online media in particular to change attitudes and to contribute to public pedagogy. They are significant in the sense that the widespread media coverage of their stories reflects and helps to shape contemporary cultural and social responses to disability in the public sphere, but also because these new kinds of photographic portraits raise ethical issues about the role of new technology and its ability to document personal experience with such immediacy and widespread accessibility. The title of Duley's 'Self-Portrait: Becoming the Story' (2011) suggests the pain, the problems, but also the possibilities for both photographers associated with this process of 'Becoming the Story'.

Action shots and autobiographical photography

Duley and Silva are contemporary photojournalists whose work focuses on capturing unrepresented stories about humanitarian issues and in sites of conflict. Throughout their careers, both men have used photography to represent disability. Duley, for example, captured the facial disfigurement of young female survivors of acid attacks in Dhaka, Bangladesh (Duley, 2009) and made a series of photos entitled 'Nick, Living with Autism' (Duley, 2006). Silva is most widely known for his membership of the Bang Bang Club: a group of photographers working in townships in South Africa to document violence and the resulting injuries during the period of transition from the Apartheid system in the early 1990s. The difficult ethical questions raised by their work, and particularly representations of disabled bodies injured in warfare, were made yet more pressing for both photographers when they were themselves injured while working as photojournalists in Afghanistan. In 2010, when on military patrol with soldiers in Kandahar, Silva stepped on a landmine and had to have both legs amputated below the knee. A year later, Duley stepped on an improvised explosive device also while on foot patrol with American soldiers and became a triple amputee, losing both of his legs and one arm.

At these moments of intense crisis, both photographers chose to turn their cameras on themselves. In an interview with the *New York Times*, Duley describes his thought process as he waited for medical aid: 'I thought, "Right hand? Eyes?" – he realized that all of these were intact – and I thought, "I can work"' (Chivers, 2011a). Later, in a 2011 exhibition in London, Duley chose to exhibit photographs of himself taken by David Bowering in the immediate aftermath of the explosion. Silva has also exhibited the photographs that he himself took moments after being injured. Released on the internet, Silva's lopsided images of earth and sky, taken from the ground as he lay incapacitated and in pain, tell a tale of terrible confusion in just three frames (Silva, 2010). Silva's commentary on these photographs echoes Duley's; they share a sense of the significance of photography as work and a commitment to documenting violence and warfare:

> Immediately [after the explosion], there were medics working on me. I picked up a camera, shot a few frames. The frames weren't very good, quite frankly, but I was trying to record. I knew it wasn't good, but I felt alive
>
> (Silva, 2011)

These action photographs create a sense of the desperate and distressing condition of the body behind the camera. Silva's commentary again catches the urgency of this human involvement and the drive to create the work:

> People tend to think there's a machine behind the camera, and that's not the case...The things that we see go through the eye straight to the brain. Some of those scenes never go away... At the other side of the camera, there is a human being, and that human being is trying to stay alive, trying to capture, trying to get the message out to the world, trying to stay safe.
>
> (Silva, 2011)

The relationship between the body and the camera becomes reconfigured here; the camera is represented not as an all-seeing eye or a protective shield, but rather as an imperfect mechanism and an extension of the body. So, Silva's focus on this moment of crisis, in which the gap between the photographer and the subject of war photographs collapses, serves as a reminder of shared human vulnerability.

These action shot portraits are not altogether new. The act of photographing a man in the moment of being wounded recalls one of the most famous and widely written about war photographs of all time: Robert Capa's 'Loyalist Militiaman at the Moment of Death, Cerro Muriano, September 5, 1936', often referred to as 'The Falling Soldier'. Capa's striking photograph, taken during the Spanish Civil War, captures the moment of death as a process, as a soldier falls backwards on a barren hillside (Capa, 2007). The photo immediately raises implicit ethical questions about the photographer's decision to persist in taking the photograph, rather than coming to the aid of the dying soldier, but also raises concerns about the safety of the photographer himself.

Duley's and Silva's photographs taken on the battlefield immediately after they were injured can be located in this tradition of action shots in photojournalism. Yet, their intensely personal focus also suggests something new in the power of modern technologies to allow access to the most intimate and troubling of moments. Duley's and Silva's images confront viewers with an overwhelming sense of immediacy: both in the ease with which a photograph can be taken following the accident, but also in terms of the ease with which these images can be disseminated and accessed worldwide through blogs and other online media. In this shift from being photographers of people with disabilities, to becoming disabled photographers, Duley and Silva self-consciously occupy positions as both passive victims of the violence of warfare and active agents in the representation of their own stories. They are insiders in the photojournalism industry and media establishment who have an intensely personal (as well as professional) interest not only in documenting stories of disability that are usually hidden from the public gaze but also in exploring the potential for photographic forms to change social attitudes toward disability.

Photography and disability theory

Since the 1990s, many disability theorists have suggested that visual representations of disability in popular culture tend to perpetuate stereotypes of Otherness, acting as symbols of helplessness, pity, and tragedy (Longmore, 1997; Garland-Thomson, 2002b; Hevey, 2013). David Hevey, in an essay included in the most recent edition of *The Disability Studies Reader* (2013), laments the dearth of nuanced photographic representations of disability and describes a wider 'enfreakment' that occurs in photographic representations of disabled people. He opens with the question: 'Apart from charity advertising, when did you last see a picture of a disabled person? It almost certainly wasn't in commercial advertising since disabled people are not thought to constitute a body of consumers' (Hevey, 2013: 432). Like Paul Longmore (1997), who has criticised many charities for perpetuating a kind of 'Tiny Tim' image of disabled vulnerability, Hevey dismisses the so-called colonisation of the bodies of people with disabilities in the representation of certain images and regrets the fact that 'disabled people are almost entirely absent from photographic genres or discussion because they are read as socially dead and not having a role to play' (Hevey, 2013: 432). For him, photography represents a repressive force of 'categorisation, control, manipulation', and public 'surveillance' in which oppressive, stereotypical attitudes toward people with disabilties are reinforced (Hevey, 2013: 445).

These anxieties about the public exploitation and surveillance of bodies deemed vulnerable are also explored in theoretical writing about photojournalism. Just as

Hevey describes the way in which photographic conventions often position people with disabilities as the 'voyeuristic property of the non-disabled gaze' (Hevey, 2013: 444), Susan Sontag, in *Regarding the Pain of Others*, explores the self-reflexive concern that we 'are voyeurs, whether or not we mean to be' (Sontag, 2004: 38). She too suggests that photography can have a metaphorically prosthetic function (Mitchell and Snyder, 2000), in the sense that it acts as a reductive, stereotypical shorthand that substitutes for informed political debate and forms a 'species of rhetoric' that reiterates, simplifies, agitates, and creates the illusion of consensus (Sontag, 2004: 5). To read *exclusively* in pictures, Sontag warns, is potentially to confirm 'a general abhorrence of war' (Sontag, 2004: 8) that leads to a sense of disengagement, as history and politics are cut out of the photographic frame.

In some ways, media coverage of the stories of Duley and Silva immediately following their accidents reinforced these stereotypical attitudes toward disability. The motif of the 'narrative of overcoming' (Garland-Thomson, 2002a: 20) – a sentimental and saleable representation of disability – is played out in certain journalistic reports of their rehabilitation. A subtitle in *The New York Times*, for example, offered a triumphalist if reductive version of Silva's story:

> Photojournalist João Silva lost his legs to a land mine in Afghanistan at the end of last year, but – after months of intense rehabilitation – returned to work in July, landing a photo on the front page of the *New York Times*
>
> (Zhang, 2011)

Alongside this account were a series of conventional 'photocall' shots of Silva with Joe Biden and Michelle Obama, in which Silva was invariably positioned passively as a patient on a hospital bed. In this narrative, Silva's privileged new role as a White House press photographer after the accident marks the culmination of a 'recovery'. The 'months of intense rehabilitation' are relegated to a brief aside, in the chronological narrative of progress and overcoming:

Dossier: João Silva
Oct. 23: He's Wounded
Oct. 26: Prescient Words
Oct. 26: Progress Reports
Nov. 29: His Last Pictures
Jan. 19: First Field Trip
Feb. 8: Taking Steps
May 5: Recording History
May 31: With the First Lady
July 28: On Page One

> (Chivers, 2011b)

Similarly, the title and publicity surrounding Channel 4's high profile documentary about Duley, called 'The Walking Wounded' (aired on prime-time television in the United Kingdom in March 2013) suggests a conventional narrative of overcoming through its dramatic emphasis on his decision to return to what was dubbed 'the scene of the crime'.

Rehabilitation portraits and self-portraits: public and private selves

In contrast to these often reductive textual narratives, many of the photographs – both of and by – Duley and Silva following their accidents offer a more nuanced exploration of their own stories and the experiences of people injured during warfare. On *The New York Times* 'Lens' blog for example, choreographed, professional images of Silva with politicians were presented alongside intimate personal portraits of the everyday experience of disability and the slow process of rehabilitation. These highly personal portraits challenge stereotypical attitudes described by Hevey and Longmore in the sense that Silva is positioned as an active participant at the centre of the frame: taking his first steps on his new prosthetic legs, but also performing everyday tasks such as getting dressed in the morning, going to a department store to buy a new shirt, or simply walking up the stairs. Through the form of the blog, Silva's life as a disabled man is presented not as a static portrait, but rather a series of snapshots of various public and private selves. This use of online media makes possible a new documentary form in which textual narratives and photographs are placed in dialogue with one another and portraits change over time. In the photographs, Silva refuses to be positioned as a passive object of the gaze. The blog as a form encourages viewers actively to return to the photographs as they are added to and updated. The dynamism of the form allows the viewer to review a narrative that remains provisional and evolving.

In a particularly powerful portrait, Silva is depicted examining himself in the mirror, confronting his new body head-on as he gets dressed for work with his prosthetic limbs on full display. The binary between viewer and viewed is destabilised as the process of looking becomes the subject of the photograph. Within this single photographic frame, Silva's body is doubled: we see his front in the mirror and his back closest to the camera. The portrait is at once distinctly modern, inserted in its particular contemporary American context through Silva's state of the art prosthetic legs, yet is also clearly situated within the long tradition of doubling and mirroring in photographic and painted portraiture that stretches from van Eyck through Rembrandt to the modern day (Rideal, 2001).

Duley, in his 'Self-Portrait: Becoming the Story' (2011), also brings together art history and activism to make a striking aesthetic as well as political statement about the power of photography to challenge problematic social attitudes toward disability through the public display of his disabled body. Selected for display at the Taylor Wassing Exhibition at London's National Portrait Gallery in 2012, the self-portrait depicts Duley without his prosthetic arms or legs in starkly contrasting black and grey. As in the portrait of Silva, the image highlights the act of looking: positioned on a plinth, Duley stares defiantly straight back at the camera. Duley actively recalls the Venus de Milo, a work of art that, Tobin Siebers suggests, is 'called beautiful by the tradition of modern aesthetic response, and yet ... eschews the uniformity of perfect bodies to embrace the variety of disability' (Siebers,

2006: 65). So, in setting up the photograph, Duley self-consciously merged the 'broken statue' image of Greek sculpture with the very contemporary fashion photography on which he himself worked early in his career: 'I wanted to ... shoot myself in the same way I'd shoot someone for Vogue. I was exactly the same person inside, but people talked to me differently because I was in a wheelchair' (Duley, 2012). Like other contemporary re-workings of the Venus de Milo image such as Marc Quinn's 'Alison Lapper, Pregnant' (2005), the disabled body is depicted as both aesthetically and physically productive; Duley uses aesthetics to challenge expectations, combining traditions from popular culture and high art to insist that viewers confront issues of disability and representation head on.

The aesthetic strategies of these portraits, which emphasise beauty, pride, and disability, can be aligned with Siebers's notion of 'disability aesthetics' as that which 'refuses to recognize the representation of the healthy body – and its definition of harmony, integrity, and beauty – as the sole determination of the aesthetic' (Siebers, 2006: 64). They mark an interesting connection between the genre of photojournalism and more traditional artistic portraits.

This connection challenges the notion that photographic representations of bodies injured in war are more rightly the subjects of photojournalism than art, and that the aesthetic treatment of the subject should therefore be documentary, captured quickly and expressive of the brutality of war. For some commentators, speed and an absence of beauty are seen as markers of authenticity; in this view, the process of aestheticisation is seen as dangerous. Susie Linfield, for example, writing on photojournalism and human rights, considers the view that:

> Photographs that depict suffering shouldn't be beautiful, as captions shouldn't moralize. In this view, a beautiful photograph drains attention from the sobering subject and turns it toward the medium itself, thereby compromising the picture's status as a document.
>
> (Linfield, 2010: 68)

By contrast, it is the assurance and exactitude with which Duley's and Silva's photographic portraits are set up that create such a powerful effect. Their self-reflexive focus on the 'medium itself' does not detract from the subject, but rather acknowledges the act of looking as a highly significant social process. Instead of a conventional caricature of victimhood or overcoming, the images depict every day, embodied experience in forms that address issues of cultural invisibility.

The more recent works produced by Duley and Silva and the widespread media coverage that they have attracted mark a wider shift toward participatory practices in contemporary photojournalism in the United States and the United Kingdom. If, as Hevey suggests, historically, 'the entire discourse has absented the voice of disabled people' (Hevey, 2013: 435) then Duley and Silva's work is important not just because it tells their own stories, but also because through it, they seek to change attitudes toward people with disabilities who are less famous than themselves.

Duley's self-portrait certainly forms part of his wider work to raise awareness about stories and experiences of disability through photography. His first job as a photographer after his accident brought his personal concerns together with a wider public interest in the United Kingdom and worldwide in the changing relationships between technology and the body. In 2012, using his own specially crafted prosthetic arm and a range of specialised tools, Duley created a series of photographs for BBC news online, depicting the technicians and prosthetists working at the London Paralympics. In October 2012, Duley returned to Afghanistan and in March 2013 photographs from his visit were exhibited in the KK Outlet Gallery in London. The fact that some of the photos featured both in the exhibition and on popular news websites suggests an intersection between different modes of display, as well as between the roles that Duley continues to play as a professional photojournalist and an advocate for disability rights. These 2012 photographs are, significantly, not of frontline soldiers, but are taken at a medical centre for civilian amputees in Kabul, run by foreign aid agencies. The photographs depict states of pain and fear during medical procedures but also, like the rehabilitation portraits of Silva, they capture moments of waiting, boredom, frustration, family intimacy, and discussions between Duley and patients in the unit. One of the most striking aspects of these images of dialogue between the photographer and the photographed is the gap that is revealed between the sophistication of the western healthcare and technology available to Duley – from his camera to his specially customised prosthetic limbs – and the meagre resources available to the small percentage of landmine victims who are actually able to make it to the hospital in Kabul. In the television documentary, Duley explicitly connects the narratives of these individual photographs to the on-going and under-represented story of the estimated 55,000 amputees and their families in Afghanistan (Duley, 2013a). Like Duley, Silva has also underlined the importance of continuing his work in war zones, to document untold stories through his photography: 'I'm a historian with a camera, and hopefully my pictures use the medium to capture history, or to tell a story, or to highlight someone else's suffering. That's ultimately why I continue doing it, and why I want to continue doing it'. (Silva, 2011)

The presence of a disabled photographer both behind and in front of the camera raises important questions about empathy. Lord Ashdown, himself a former soldier, celebrated Duley's Afghanistan photographs for their ability to 'remind us of our humanity and the need for understanding and compassion' (Duley, 2013b). The photographs raise questions about the means through which contemporary media can tell stories and change attitudes among wider, international audiences through individualised, local snapshots or portraits. In this context, notions of 'intercorporeality' taken up in disability studies (Paterson and Hughes, 1999: 604) intersect with arguments made by human rights activists about the power of photography in the modern world. Linfield has suggested:

> The very thing that critics have assailed photographs for *not* doing – explaining causation, process, relationships – is connected to the very thing they do so

well: present us, to ourselves and each other, as bodily creatures ... Photographs show how easily we are reduced to the merely physical ... The vulnerability is something that every human being shares.

(Linfield, 2010: 68)

Even in her critique of photojournalism, Sontag echoes this sense of the potentially democratising power of photography to promote visual storytelling in an accessible way: 'In contrast to a written account – which, depending on its complexity of thought, reference, and vocabulary, is pitched at a larger or smaller readership – a photograph has only one language and is destined for all' (Sontag, 2004: 17).

Yet, the accessible nature of photographs in contemporary culture does not mean that they can be easily 'read', not least because of the shifting expectations that viewers bring to images depending on whether they are presented as historical documents, aesthetic objects, or transient reportage. Recently, critics have begun to suggest that the borrowing of literary critical vocabularies, in which photography is conceived of as a visual language, needs to be replaced with a more sophisticated 'intermedial' criticism that acknowledges the exchange between words and images in the age of new media (Louvel, 2008: 44; Siebers, 2010: 133). In the work of Duley and Silva, the dynamism of the exchange between text and image on their blogs and in their exhibitions creates a new form of portraiture. The interplay between Duley's and Silva's roles as photojournalists, artists, civilians, and private citizens creates a new role for the self-portraitist.

Conclusion: public pedagogies and popular culture

There are dangers in idealising the power of photographic images, or other cultural forms, to bring about changes in cultural and social attitudes. Yet, this is an active area in both practical and theoretical terms. The explosion in 'citizen journalism' organisations such as 'Photovoice', for example, uses photography to try to address issues of voicelessness among marginalised groups including people with disabilities, through projects that offer free training in the use of basic equipment. They acknowledge the potential for photographs to stigmatise certain groups by identifying them as vulnerable, but they are informed by creative, participatory aesthetics and practices that have only recently become possible through new media. In the age of the image, such organisations assert the importance of the practice of photography in raising awareness and public education. As Henri Giroux points out, 'pedagogy is rarely taken up as part of a broader public politics' but there is enormous potential in 'assess[ing] the political significance of understanding the broader educational force of culture in the new age of media technology, multimedia, and computer-based information and communication networks' (Giroux, 2004: 60). Duley's and Silva's work self-consciously exploits the potential of photography as a public pedagogy intended to promote more varied representations and better understanding about disability issues in the United Kingdom, the United States, and beyond. Their portraits place living, changing disabled bodies at the centre of the frame; their autobiographical texts and images highlight the role of the human body of the photographer behind the camera but also the active, embodied role of viewers interpreting the picture. In this context, the active, participatory process of teaching, assessing and interpreting these images becomes an important activity in itself, not only for documenting changing attitudes toward disability, but also for bringing social change. Cases such as those of Duley and Silva, where the photographer becomes the story, have something to teach us beyond the individual: they particularise experience and, like a camera, provide a lens through which to focus on a wider set of issues about empathy, online media, and the need for more complex and diverse representations of disability in twenty-first century culture.

References

Capa, R. (2007) Loyalist militiaman at the moment of death, Cerro Muriano, 5 September. 1936. 9 July. Online. Available http://photo.net/black-and-white-photo-printing-finishing-forum/00LoAu (accessed 15 August 2013).

Chivers, C.J. (2011a) Bomb took 3 limbs, but not photographer's can-do spirit. 8 July. Online. Available www.nytimes.com/2011/07/09/world/europe/09duley.html?ref=science (accessed 15 August 2013).

Chivers, C.J. (2011b) A test, and gratitude, at the Whitehouse. 15 September. Online. Available http://lens.blogs.nytimes.com/2011/09/15/joao-silva-at-the-white-house/ (accessed 15 August 2013).

Duley, G. (2006) Nick, living with autism. Online. Available http://gilesduley.com/#/galleries/nick-living-with-autism-2006/website-11 (accessed 15 August 2013).

Duley, G. (2009) Acid burn survivors, Dhaka, Bangladesh. Online. Available http://gilesduley.com/#/galleries/acid-burn-survivors-dhaka-bangladesh-2009/acidburnsrevisions_4 (accessed 15 August 2013).

Duley, G. (2011) Becoming the story: self-portrait. Online. Available http://gilesduley.com/#/galleries/becoming-the-story-self-portrait-london-2011/self-portrait_2 (accessed 15 August 2013).

Duley, G. (2012) BBC interview. September. Online. Available http://gilesduley.com/#/interviews/bbc-news-magazine--sep-2012 (accessed 15 August 2013).

Duley, G. (2013a) Walking wounded: The return to the front line. 21 February. Online. Available www.channel4.com/programmes/walking-wounded-return-to-the-frontline (accessed 15 August 2013).

Duley, G. (2013b) Bio. Online. Available http://gilesduley.com/#/bio (accessed 15 August 2013).

Garland-Thomson, R. (2002a) Integrating disability, transforming feminist theory. *NWSA Journal*, 14, 3, 1–32.

Garland-Thomson, R. (2002b) The politics of staring: visual rhetorics of disability in popular photography', in S.L. Snyder, B.J Brueggeman, and R. Garland-Thomson (eds) *Disability Studies: Enabling the Humanities*, New York: Modern Language Association of America.

Giroux, H.A. (2004) Cultural studies, public pedagogy and the responsibility of intellectuals, *Communication and Critical / Cultural Studies*, 1, 1, 59–79.

Hevey, D. (2013) The enfreakment of photography, in L.J. Davis (ed.) *The Disability Studies Reader*, London: Routledge.

Hocks, M.E. and Kendrick, M.R. (2005) *Eloquent Images: Word and Image in the Age of New Media*, Cambridge: MIT Press.

Linfield, S. (2010) *The Cruel Radiance: Photography and Political Violence*, Chicago: Chicago University Press.

Longmore, P.K. (1997) Conspicuous contribution and American cultural dilemmas: telethon rituals of cleansing and renewal, in D.T. Mitchell and S.L. Snyder (eds) *The Body and Physical Difference: Discourses of Disability in the Humanities*, Ann Arbor: University of Michigan Press.

Louvel, L. (2008) Photography as critical idiom and intermedial criticism, *Poetics Today*, 29, 1, 31–48.

Mitchell, D.T. and Snyder, S.L. (2000) *Narrative Prosthesis: Disability and the Dependencies of Discourse*, Ann Arbor: University of Michigan Press.

Paterson, K. and Hughes, B. (1999) Disability studies and phenomenology, *Disability and Society*, 14, 597–601.

Rideal, L. (ed.) (2001) *Mirror Mirror: Self-portraits by Women Artists*, London: National Portrait Gallery.

Sontag, S. (2004) *Regarding the Pain of Others*, London: Penguin.

Siebers, T. (2010) *Disability Aesthetics*, Ann Arbor: University of Michigan Press.

Siebers, T. (2006) Disability aesthetics, *JCRT*, 7, 2, 63–73.

Silva, J. (2010) Joao Silva for The New York Times. 23 October. Online. Available http://digiphotomag.com/wp-content/uploads/Joao-Silva_NYT.png (accessed 15 August 2013).

Silva, J. (2011) This is what I do. This is all that I know. August 30. Online. Available http://lens.blogs.nytimes.com/2011/08/30/this-is-what-i-do-this-is-all-that-i-know/ (accessed 15 August 2013).

Zhang, M. (2011) Photojournalist Joao Silva on life, loss and conflict photography. 30 August. Online. Available http://petapixel.com/2011/08/30/photojournalist-joao-silva-on-life-loss-and-conflict-photography/ (accessed 15 August 2013).

5 Mental disability and rhetoricity retold

The memoir on drugs

Catherine Prendergast

More than a decade ago in a chapter for the volume *Embodied Rhetorics: Disability in Language and Culture*, I wrote, 'To be disabled mentally is to be disabled rhetorically' (Prendergast, 2001: 57). I am writing this chapter to un-write that one. I argued in 'On the Rhetorics of Mental Disability' that bearing a diagnosis of a mental disorder compromised a rhetor's position generally, and with extra force in institutional contexts such as the clinician's office, prison, or the court. My case was built largely upon a memoir – my own – recounting my relationship with Barbara, a woman with schizophrenia. The period of time the memoir covered included recollections from the 1990s, an era during which a new class of antipsychotic drugs was just emerging, drugs that would materially change living circumstances for many people with schizophrenia, including Barbara. These drugs have also significantly altered the rhetorical conditions of people with schizophrenia. Since the 1990s, several publications have emerged featuring the work of authors self-identifying as having experienced psychosis, including *SZ Magazine, New York City Voices*, and *Shift Journal*. This same time period marks the beginning of a wave of published memoirs by authors self-identifying as having psychiatric impairments. Each of these works engages the issue of living, working, and writing with a mental disability. Collectively they demonstrate that what I wrote in my short memoir – that to be disabled mentally is to be disabled rhetorically – was wrong. What I write here as I revisit the issue, then, could be considered a long form *mea culpa*.

First, I must acknowledge those numerous colleagues in the corner of disability studies concerned with rhetoric who were more thoughtful than I was. Cynthia Lewiecki-Wilson, for example, has argued that in considerations of disability and rhetoricity, a 'sharp demarcation between individual rhetorical agency and its lack' is to be avoided (Lewiecki-Wilson, 2013: 162). She envisioned instances where speech is co-constructed with parents, care-givers, or through technological means. Such moments of mediated communication should, she argued rightly, count as instances of exercising rhetorical agency. Janell Johnson has similarly called for an expanded notion of rhetoricity (Johnson, 2010). She has highlighted the contingent nature of *ethos* as it is dependent on situation, time, and place. She argued that qualities that bolstered a rhetor's *ethos* in one situation might degrade that *ethos* in another. Because rhetorical agency is ever-shifting in time, we cannot come to an assessment as to degree of rhetorical agency by looking at one point in history, or even one point in a life history.

Katie Rose Guest Pryal addresses the shortcomings of my approach on madness and rhetoricity most directly, however, as she argues for the rhetorical force and artistry of memoirs written by authors with mood disorders (Guest Pryal, 2010). She argues that my assertion 'to be disabled mentally is to be disabled rhetorically' fails to recognise how people who are mentally disabled might claim rhetorical agency through several sources, including the Platonic equation of poetry with divine madness (Guest Pryal, 2010: 482). Her analysis of memoirists of mood disorders effectively demonstrates that authority is often claimed *because* and not *despite* of the presence of a diagnosis. She outlines four rhetorical moves characteristic of the 'mood memoir': an *apologia* that gives reasons for writing the memoir; a 'moment of awakening' to the mental illness; a criticism of 'bad' doctors; and *auxesis*, through which the ability to speak for others with the same impairment is claimed (Guest Pryal, 2010: 485).

My concern is and always has been the writing of those diagnosed with schizophrenia, a condition that Guest Pryal notes she excluded from consideration when bounding her project around the memoir written by people diagnosed with a mood disorder. Nevertheless, the rhetorical gestures of the mood disorder memoir she identifies map *almost* seamlessly onto the schizophrenia memoir. In this chapter I explore the specific features of two memoirs written recently by schizophrenics and read widely: Ken Steele's *The Day the Voices Stopped* (2001) and Elyn Saks's *The Center Cannot Hold* (2007). These memoirs were far and away not the first publications of either author. Steele had been since 1995 editor and staff writer in the magazine for mental health consumers that he founded, *New York City Voices*. Saks, endowed professor of law and psychiatry at the University of Southern California, had published articles and books related to her area of scholarship, the rights of people who are mentally ill. Steele unfortunately died before the publication of his life story, making his memoir his exiting, rather than entering, work in the public arena. Saks has been able to widen her role as spokesperson beyond the memoir. In June 2012, she made perhaps the most public of rhetorical gestures: She gave a TED talk.

The memoirs of Steele and Saks feature many of the rhetorical gestures Guest Pryal identified in her analysis of the mood memoir. Both Steele and Saks testify in their writing to the appalling standard of care they experienced in the United States, and to their desire to improve that standard. Yet both also acknowledge the necessity of medication and treatment as means toward maintaining their relationships, activism, and professional lives. Their faith in the psychiatric profession and appropriate psychopharmacology is expressed in their memoirs despite the lengthy descriptions of their experiences with abusive hospital conditions, stressed or under-informed doctors, and ineffective medicine. Their memoirs are just as much affirmations of 'good' doctors and effective medical intervention as they are critiques of 'bad' doctors and failed treatments.

The memoir on drugs

Bearing this tension in mind, here I argue that the main rhetorical task of the memoir written by an author with schizophrenia is to reckon with the complexity of drugs and society rather than to indict the medical model wholesale. The memoirs of Steele and Saks organise around the moment in which they accepted, rather than resisted, drug therapy. After this moment, their memoirs both chart a narrative arc toward productivity, public activism, and mended relationships. The memoir of the person with schizophrenia is, then, a 'memoir on drugs' in all ways: it is a memoir written while the author is on drugs, but it is also a memoir *on* the subject of drugs, and their value, their history, their life in the social imagination. Drugs are, according to the memoirist, a large part of why they can tell their story at all.

This rhetorical work of the memoir on drugs seems difficult for disability studies, as so much energy to date has been devoted to crafting a (needed) critique of the medical model. Guest Pryal's analysis of the mood memoir concludes, for example, that 'the mood memoir should be seen as a counter-narrative to a dominant narrative of mental illness put forward by the psychiatric profession' (Guest Pryal, 2010: 483). I have found, however, those who are part and parcel of the psychiatric profession (e.g., psychiatrists Jamison and Saks), and also grateful beneficiaries of it (e.g., Jamison, Saks, and Steele), are just as likely in their memoirs to extol the psychiatric profession. Kay Redfield Jamison's *An Unquiet Mind*, for example, argues for the medical treatment of mental illness as rigorously as it lodges complaints against 'bad' doctors (Jamison, 1995). The memoirs of people who are mentally ill are not so much concerned with a wholesale indictment of psychiatry as with countering the prevailing myths that mental illness does not exist or cannot be humanely treated. Ultimately, the 'memoir on drugs' forms a counter-narrative not to the psychiatric profession, but to the anti-psychiatry movement. It establishes political voice, productivity, and public activism on other grounds than a rejection of psychiatry. In short, the task of the memoir on drugs is to work through an initially conflicted, but eventually resolved understanding of the medical understanding of schizophrenia.

The problem with chemical straightjackets

In the memoir of physical disability, it is the wheelchair, not medication, which takes center stage as the material object with which to be reckoned. Through the memoir on physical disability, the wheelchair must be refigured: portrayed by ableism to be the symbol of restraint and loss, it is recast as a means to freedom and mark of identity. Thus the late Harriet McBryde Johnson in her 'Unspeakable Conversations' recalls having to educate onlookers who pity her for being in a wheelchair, 'It's a great sensual pleasure to zoom by power chair on these delicious muggy streets' (McBryde Johnson, 2013: 509). Simi Linton transforms her wheelchair into a 'sidekick' named Rufus. Linton and Rufus often go to the Guggenheim Museum, which is refigured in her narrative as 'a wheelchair-pleasing building' (Linton, 2007: 187). In her epilogue, she considers a child – real or dreamt, she is not sure – who considers her wheelchair not a fearsome sign of dread, but a carnival ride.

Linton's and McBryde Johnson's memoirs both seek to refigure the rhetorical work that wheelchairs do in the world: from symbol of constraint, to symbol of freedom of expression and movement. Interestingly, both memoirs also mention drugs, but largely in passing. McBryde Johnson acknowledges that her life would have been impossible without medication. She writes, 'I am in the first generation to survive to such decrepitude. Because antibiotics were available, we didn't die from the childhood pneumonias that often come with weakened respiratory systems' (McBryde Johnson, 2013: 508). She acknowledges that without the medication, she would not have lived to be in a wheelchair at all. Linton's memoir does not detail the role of antibiotics or other drugs in saving her life after her accident, though they almost certainly were used, but she does mention substantial other medical equipment. There are drugs mentioned in *My Body Politic*, however they are of a recreational nature – a mark of identity and expression (Linton, 2007). Neither McBryde Johnson nor Linton are dis-qualified from full participation in the disability rights movement due to their drug use; each has been a foremost speaker for the rights of people with disabilities.

Discussion of the role of antipsychotic medication in the treatment of people who are mentally ill, however, immediately forces one into conflict with the anti-psychiatry or 'Mad Pride' movement, which claims the civil rights movement as its inspiration for fighting the psychiatry profession's oppression of people who are mentally ill. The anti-psychiatry movement does genuinely provide a counter-narrative to the medical model of mental illness. In 2003, for example, MindFreedom International (MFI), an active organisation in the anti-psychiatry movement, staged a 25-day hunger strike to force the American Psychiatric Association (APA), the National Alliance for the Mentally Ill, or the Surgeon General to provide scientific evidence of the biological basis for mental illness (MFI, 2013). Among these groups, the APA was the only one to respond, sending citations from scientific journals (MFI's Science Advisory Board considered these upon review to be insufficient evidence). MFI (previously known as Support Coalition International) is careful to distinguish itself from the Citizen's Commission on Human Rights (CCHR) co-founded by Thomas Szasz and the Church of Scientology in 1969. While a minority of mental health consumers identify with either of these organisations, the broader cultural milieu has absorbed the rhetoric of the anti-psychiatry movement. A Google search I conducted in August of 2013 on the phrase that Szasz popularised, 'chemical straightjackets', returns over 62,000 hits (even when controlled for the name of a rock band of the same name – though the fact that 'chemical straightjackets' is a band name, and thus 'cool,' is itself interesting).

As Susan Sontag reminds us, clichés such as 'chemical straightjackets' have social force (Sontag, 2011). Remarking on the problematic associations that are attached to cancer or AIDS through metaphors, she has argued, 'It is highly desirable for a specific dreaded illness to come to be seen as ordinary ... Much in the way of individual experience and social policy depends on the struggle for rhetorical ownership of the illness: how it is possessed, assimilated in argument and in cliché' (Sontag, 2011: 182). Just as the memoir written by those with physical impairments must refigure the wheelchair as enabling rather than restraining, the memoir on drugs must confront a history of suspicion of antipsychotic medication and refigure drugs as useful.

Steele's memoir describes in great detail, for example, the moment his voices stopped following a course of Risperdal. He recalls having felt so bombarded by the unfamiliar sounds of the outside world that he stayed curled up in his bathtub for three days. Following his initial shock, however, he describes the freedom that cessation of psychosis had brought: 'For the first time in decades, I was free to hear the voices of others, even when they weren't speaking to or about me' (Steele, 2001: 202). He describes that when his psychiatrist had initially suggested he try the new medication, he had been unwilling, given his experience with ineffective courses of treatment in the past. Only after he is sure that his voices have truly gone does he admit to his psychiatrist that the treatment is working. He pens a letter of gratitude to his doctor: 'Thank you for convincing me to try this medication. You didn't lie to me. The side effects are minimal. You've given me back my life. I don't know what I'm going to do with it, but you've given me a second chance' (Steele, 2001: 205). The rhetorical work Steele does of walking the reader through his moment of accepting medication is so significant that he titled his memoir *The Day the Voices Stopped*.

Saks similarly devotes much of her memoir to recounting her evolving attitude toward medication. She describes that her initial debilitating fears of psychiatric medication began with her mis-diagnosis as a drug addict when she was a teenager. She had been taught that will power, not chemicals, would solve all her problems. When it was first suggested she take an anti-depressant, she rejected the idea: 'Pills? Something chemical to go into my body and muck about with it? No, that would be wrong' (Saks, 2007: 58). Only the certainty that she would kill herself if she did not try medication brings her to the moment where she does take pills that not only pull her out of depression but also allow her to concentrate on her studies at Oxford. Yet her anti-drug stance remains to the extent that getting off them becomes her persistent goal, with the result that psychosis returns again and again. Finally, Saks, like Steele, tries one of the class of atypical antipsychotic medications that emerged in the 1990s, and she experiences what she refers to as the most convincing argument that she had ever been presented that she indeed had a mental illness: 'The most profound effect of the new drug was to convince me, once and for all, that I actually had a real illness. For twenty years, I'd struggled with that acceptance, coming right up to it on some days, backing away from it on most others. The clarity that Zyprexa gave me knocked down my last remaining argument' (Saks, 2007: 304). She discovers that the more she accepts her diagnosis, the less it, and the illness it names, defines her. To return to Guest Pryal's framework of significant rhetorical turns of the memoir, we might say the 'moment of awakening' to mental illness in Saks's memoir is enabled by the drug (Guest Pryal, 2010: 485). The drug had both material and rhetorical effect. The drug, as Saks recalled, persuaded her that she was ill, and then allowed her to resume her work articulating the difference between humane and abusive treatment of mentally ill people.

The memoirs of Saks and Steele are both unsparing in their depictions of psychiatric abuse. Steele was restrained, beaten, raped, and forcefully medicated with mind-numbing and ineffective drugs while in a psychiatric institution. Saks's memoir chronicles her experience with bad doctors as well as good ones. She is careful to draw a distinction in her memoir between medication she is persuaded to try and the situation of 'being tied to a bed against your will and force-fed medication you did not ask for and do not understand' (Saks, 2007: 331). Both these memoirs are clear on the point that to be in a straightjacket, to be forcibly restrained, is an entirely different experience than being on effective psychosis-relieving medication that one has elected to take. In her TED talk, Saks most brightly draws the distinction between treatment and abuse of people who are mentally disabled when she announces, 'I am pro-psychiatry, and anti-force' (Saks, 2012). With this statement, Saks neatly cleaves the persistent metaphor of the 'chemical straightjacket'. She identifies herself as pro-chemical, but anti-straightjacket. The memoirs of both Saks and Steele refigure medications – from restraints to liberators – in much the same way as Linton's and McBryde Johnson's memoirs refigured the wheelchair. 'Chemical wheelchairs' might be a more accurate metaphor for capturing the role of antipsychotic medication in the memoir on drugs. A Google search under 'chemical wheelchairs', however, yields only 77 hits (far fewer than the 62,000 for 'chemical straightjackets'); most of these hits take the reader to links related to the use of chemicals in wheelchairs.

But perhaps it is best to avoid metaphoric thinking altogether (Sontag, 2011). Antipsychotics are, like antibiotics, just another chemical. It is probably better, then, just to think of anti-psychotic medication as just anti-psychotic medication, and to believe those who offer their experience of taking it. In her TED talk, Saks seems to eschew metaphors, identifying herself clinically and directly, as 'a woman with chronic schizophrenia', which she terms simply as 'a brain disease' (Saks, 2012). She explains that schizophrenia should not be confused with the metaphorical use of the term, suggesting multiple personalities. Perhaps owing to the genre of the TED talk, her tone is spare and literal. She does not suggest that she is cured. She does not suggest that she wants to get off medication. Her memoir suggests that rather than discuss 'medication' as an absolute good or ill, it would be useful to recognise that there are different medications, different contexts of its use, and different effects for different people. I believe her greatest accomplishment, and Steele's, is to remind us that we should not be concerned with establishing whether drugs are good or bad, but should instead concern ourselves with the humans, including ourselves, who use them.

Life as adaptation

The impact of atypical antipsychotics on the shape of public writing by people with diagnoses of schizophrenia might one day be credited with being as significant for our larger culture as the advent of the birth control pill was for the feminist movement. Psychiatric medications have returned people to their professional lives, and allowed for this explosion of writing that documents the experience of psychosis – and ensuing relief from it – from the inside. Medication is part and parcel of other accommodations that should be considered rights of people who are mentally disabled.

In her TED talk, Saks credits her success (yes, she uses the word success quite often, though chiefly to describe her greatest accomplishment as having avoided hospitalisation for thirty years) to political and social changes brought by the disability rights movement (Saks, 2012). In a refusal to see these factors enabling her success as necessarily opposing the medical intervention of psychiatric treatment, she mentions treatment as number one on her list: 'First, I've had excellent treatment and excellent pharmacology' (Saks, 2012). The two factors that follow include family friends and her employer, the University of Southern California, which she describes as 'a place that not only accommodates my needs but embraces them' (Saks, 2012). Placing medication on a par with employer and social support is a radical gesture, suggesting not a counter-narrative to the 'medical model' so much as an embrace of it. Certainly the stigma of mental illness is not banished by adding to its scariness through a broad dismissal all treatments as the equivalent of physical restraints, or by suggesting that the only rhetorical agency a person with a brain disease can claim is through adopting the role of psychiatric survivor, eschewing all medication. The rights of people who are mentally disabled include rights to effective medications with fewer side effects, insurance parity, elevated standards of care, and other markers of humane treatment – not simply the absence of physical restraints.

From a pragmatic standpoint, any wholesale dismissal of the historic fact of widely effective medication renders us unable to intervene in social and policy discussions over its uses – and abuses. As Elizabeth Donaldson has cogently argued in her critique of the 'madness as rebellion' trope, it is possible to understand mental illness as a neurobiological disorder, and still be committed to disability studies (Donaldson, 2002). Like Donaldson, I believe the anti-psychiatry movement has been unappreciated as a 'sanist' movement, one that fails to recognise the many who are pro-psychiatry advocates for the rights of people who are mentally ill. The singling out of anti-psychotic medication for protest by the anti-psychiatry movement is particularly invidious, as it misses the fact that we are all on drugs pretty much all the time. Drugs enable all our work, from the ibuprofen that a factory worker takes to relieve a backache, to the insulin a diabetic takes to maintain her or his blood sugar level, to the caffeine I drink to help me meet a deadline for an article. It is the worst kind of sanism/ablism, to suggest that those with a diagnosis of mental disability alone should abstain from drugs, should be held to a state purified from drug use in order to be considered credible as disability rights advocates.

Conclusion

Saks wrote in her 2013 *New York Times* Op-Ed, 'People underestimate the power of the human brain to adapt and to create' (Saks, 2013). I am one of those people. I now look at that sentence I wrote many years ago – 'to be disabled mentally is to be disabled rhetorically' (Prendergast, 2001) – as worse than a faulty claim: It was a flawed prognosis, one that underestimated both the schizophrenic rhetor and the psychiatric establishment that has discovered more effective, if always imperfect, medications. I had failed to imagine anything further than the social barriers that could never be overcome by the artfulness of the schizophrenic rhetor. Now I read 'to be disabled mentally is to be disabled rhetorically' as something like the equivalent of, 'Well, there's nothing *wrong* with [homosexuality, inter-racial marriage, adopting, being on a respirator] just that it will be so very, very difficult to live with'. The point of scholarship, I hope, is not only to change the attitudes of others, but also to allow our own attitudes to change. My scholarly engagement with the writing of people diagnosed with schizophrenia has led me to a deepened appreciation of their rhetorical work.

To paraphrase Saks, one should never underestimate the power of the human rhetor to adapt and create.

References

Donaldson, E.J. (2002) The corpus of a madwoman: toward a feminist disability studies theory of embodiment and mental illness, *NWSA Journal*, 14, 3, 99–119.

Guest Pryal, K.R. (2010) The genre of the mood memoir and the ethos of psychiatric disability, *Rhetoric Society Quarterly*, 40, 5, 479–501.

Johnson, H.M. (2013) Unspeakable conversations, in L.J. Davis (ed.) *Disability Studies Reader*, New York: Routledge.

Jamison, K.R. (1995) *An Unquiet Mind: A Memoir of Moods and Madness*, New York: Vintage.

Johnson, J. (2010) The skeleton on the couch: the Eagleton affair, rhetorical disability, and the stigma of mental illness, *Rhetoric Society Quarterly*, 40, 5, 459–78.

Lewiecki-Wilson, C. (2003) Rethinking rhetoric through mental disabilities, *Rhetoric Review*, 22, 2, 156.

Linton, S. (2007) *My Body Politic: A Memoir*, Ann Arbor: University of Michigan Press.

MindFreedom International. (2013) *MindFreedom.org*. Online. Available www.mindfreedom.org/kb/act/2003/mf-hunger-strike/?searchterm=hunger%20strike (accessed 14 October 2013).

Prendergast, C. (2001) On the rhetorics of mental disability, in J.C. Wilson and C. Lewiwcki-Wilson (eds) *Embodied Rhetorics: Disability in Language and Culture*, Carbondale: Southern Illinois University Press.

Saks, E.R. (2007) *The Center Cannot Hold: My Journey through Madness*, New York: Hyperion.

Saks, E.R. (2013) Successful and schizophrenic, Op-Ed, *The New York Times*, January 27, SR5.

Saks, E.R. (2012) TED Talk: A tale of mental illness – from the inside. Online. Available www.ted.com/talks/elyn_saks_seeing_mental_illness.html (accessed 14 October 2013).

Steele, K. with Berman, C. (2001) *The Day The Voices Stopped: A Memoir of Madness and Hope*, New York, Basic.

Sontag, S. (2011) *Illness as Metaphor and Aids and its Metaphors*, New York: Picador Press.

Part II
Disability, attitudes, and culture

6 The 'hunchback'

Across cultures and time

Tom Coogan

There is a historically and culturally traceable discourse of the so-called hunchback that reveals much about changing social attitudes toward disability. Accordingly, in this chapter I begin by examining the effect of the recent introduction of the 'real' spine of Richard III into the long-running debate over the king's supposed hunchback. This development serves to illustrate the power of representation to trump reality, a power that can only be understood through a thorough examination of the historical context of the figure of the hunchback and the changing attitudes toward it. In terms of approach, I argue that it is necessary to go beyond the 'history of attitudes' toward disability (Longmore, 1985), to follow the contention that the wider history of anomalous bodies can 'reveal fissures in an otherwise monolithic discourse of modernity's production of the disabled subject' (Williams, 2009). I also provide some brief examples of representations of the hunchback and suggest how they might contribute to the critical documentation of attitudes toward disability through the lens of cultural studies.

Twisting spines

'The hunchback is dead – long live Good King Richard', read the headline of Chris Skidmore's recent article for *The Telegraph* (Skidmore, 2013). In anticipation of public confirmation that Richard III's body had been found, the historian and Conservative MP sought to make the case for the real, 'good' Richard by displacing the 'bad' Richard of popular culture onto his impairment. This is the continuation of an established historical debate in the United Kingdom, as the University of Leicester's website for the excavation makes clear in its section on 'Myths and Legends'. Contemporary historical orthodoxy holds that 'all descriptions and depictions of the King as a "crookback" derived from Tudor propaganda', in an era when 'physical deformity was thought to reflect a deformed mind and evil intent' (University of Leicester, 2013). However, Tudor accounts were by no means uniform: some describe him 'as having his left shoulder higher than his right, some say the other way round, many don't mention any deformity at all' (University of Leicester, 2013). The website observes that X-ray analysis of portraits painted after Richard's death indicate alteration to match the accepted (i.e., Tudor) image of him. The website concludes, though, that 'the curved spine of the remains found at Greyfriars has reopened this debate' (University of Leicester, 2013).

Why does Richard's real spine re-open, rather than close the matter? Semantic differences and the lay appropriation of the authority of medical terminology are particularly important here. The Leicester website refers to the 'mythical' Richard as a 'crookback', and an article by Sarah Knight and Mary Ann Lund expands upon the origins of this nickname. While their attempt to pin down the origins of a term that, they observe, was used for any and all types of 'spinal abnormality and bending' is admirable (Knight and Lund, 2013), their precision is limited by their trans-historical, catch-all use of the modern term *disability* to describe what many disability studies scholars would now call impairment (i.e., Richard's physical state). They note 'how influential Shakespeare's version of Richard's body has been', yet suggest that Shakespeare's coining of the term *hunch-backed* in the second quarto of *Richard III* (1598) may have been a typographical mis-setting of *bunch-backed*, and furthermore may result from his misinterpretation of the word *crookback* in earlier accounts (Knight and Lund, 2013). They note that a seventeenth-century translation of classifications of spinal deformities by French royal surgeon Ambroise Paré distinguishes between kyphosis (a dislocated vertebra causing a 'bunching' of the spine) and scoliosis or 'crookednesse' (a sideways curvature of the spine). They reason that Richard's skeleton has 'severe scoliosis', although they do not provide the parameters for this classification (i.e., degree of curve, etc.). They argue that this scoliosis is the 'crookednesse' that prompted Richard's 'crook-back' reputation, later misinterpreted by Shakespeare as kyphosis (Knight and Lund, 2013). They are mistaken in a key assumption, however. While kyphosis causes a spine hump, thoracic scoliosis can cause a rib hump, as ribs twist out of alignment. To a casual observer, either might be a hunchback.

While acknowledging news of the curved spine as 'the most alluring clue as to the skeleton's identity', Skidmore insists upon his own image of Richard, based on accounts from the battlefield that are hundreds of years old (Skidmore, 2013). He insists that tales of Richard the 'formidable fighter' are 'hardly in keeping with his reputation as a hunchback' (Skidmore, 2013). This assumption of mutual exclusivity perhaps says more about Skidmore's assumptions than it does about Richard or the evidence to hand. These assumptions are clearly drawn from wider culture rather than his personal knowledge or experience. Nor was *The Telegraph* the only respected newspaper to experience discombobulation at the joining of myth and reality. The *Washington Post* printed a picture of the markedly curved spine of the skeleton below the headline 'Amazing photo of King Richard III's tiny, curved spine proves Shakespeare was wrong' (Fisher, 2013). Yet the writer Max Fisher argues that the skeleton means that 'the mental image you probably have of [Richard] turns out to be him' (Fisher, 2013). Fisher then, like Lund and Knight, claims, incorrectly, that scoliosis cannot cause a hunchback and blames Shakespeare's play for having 'warped our collective understanding of Richard III as sharply as his world-famous spine' (Fisher, 2013).

How can the evidence for the reality of Richard's impairment be taken as proof that he was not really impaired at all, and what is the significance of this reaction? Arguably, for all the contemporary commentators' remarks about the unenlightened Tudors and their smears, it would appear that modern society is still a place where myths about disabled people are used for political ends. The idea of disabled people as scroungers and malingerers is endlessly repeated by the right-wing press in the United Kingdom to justify government cuts, as people like Linda Wootton are 'tested' and told that they are 'fit for work' just days before their deaths. This manipulation of semantics is not limited to disability: in 2007, in the United States, *TIME Magazine* asked 'Is Obama Black Enough?' This is the trap of identity politics: those who impose an identity to disempower will not hesitate to disavow it the moment it is reclaimed as a rallying point for the oppressed. Skidmore, Fisher, Knight and Lund are, in a way, asking if Richard is 'hunchbacked enough'.

Clearly, a more careful approach, free of unconscious contemporary cultural assumptions and attitudes, is needed to examine the historical figure of the hunchback. This problem is examined in greater detail in Paul Longmore's review of Bruce Clayton's biography of Randolph Bourne. Although Bourne is broadly read as a disabled historical figure, with his facial defects and curved spine, he could also be contextualised within the history of the hunchback. Longmore argues that Clayton has a 'fundamental misunderstanding' of his subject's disability due to his ignorance of the 'history of disabled people' (Longmore, 1985: 581). He argues that social and cultural, rather than functional, barriers were Bourne's biggest problem – for example, Imagist poet Amy Lowell's dismissal of Bourne with the words 'His writing shows he is a cripple ... Deformed body, deformed mind' (Longmore, 1985: 583). He argues that Clayton's text not only fails to examine this social and cultural element, but also, albeit unconsciously, is itself tainted by such attitudes, as apparent in the usage of 'prejudiced and highly offensive' terms such as *deformed, misshapen,* and *cripple* (Longmore, 1985: 585–86). Bourne himself carefully avoided these terms, revising his noted essay 'The Handicapped' (1911) to remove the word *deformed* (Longmore, 1985: 585–86). Longmore stresses the need to 'study literary and artistic images of disabled people and descriptions of individuals like Bourne in order to uncover cultural beliefs', to trace a 'history of ... attitudes', the better to understand the social history of disability (Longmore, 1985: 586).

Longmore's approach is a great improvement, but is arguably limited by the porous and historically specific nature of *disability* as a category. This point is explored by Katherine Schaap Williams in her work on *Richard III.* She emphasises the danger of conflating 'disability' with what she calls 'the language of deformity' (Williams, 2009). She argues that, for disability studies, 'disability' emerges after the Renaissance, in tandem with a medicalising discourse that 'classifies, regulates, and constructs bodies as "normal" or "abnormal"' (Williams, 2009). Reading a Renaissance text from this perspective, she insists, 'obscures the complexity of Richard's bodily signification by assuming a unified discourse of deformity that maps onto physical disability' (Williams, 2009).

History of the hunchback

I aim to sidestep the problem identified by Williams by focusing on a particular figure to form a tighter, more cohesive category, while simultaneously acknowledging the strategic nature of that category. There is a historically traceable discourse of the hunchback. This history of cultural representation both pre-exists and informs modern notions of disability. A full account of it would fill a book, so the points mentioned here are intended simply to highlight some areas for future research. The history of the hunchback runs from ancient history to present day, and across cultures, sometimes as a marginal figure, sometimes as a central one. This history has yet to be viewed in its proper context from the unified perspective that cultural disability studies can offer. From the *Iliad* to animated Disney features, from canonical works to more obscure representations, there is a variety of hunchbacks to be linked together. Nor has culture been shaped solely by fictional hunchbacks: the work of figures such as parliamentarian William Hay, poet Alexander Pope, and intellectuals Randolph Bourne and Antonio Gramsci has informed, just as it has been informed by, the cultures that give the figure of the hunchback its modern meaning – but has seldom been understood in its appropriate context.

As already shown, Richard III looms large in the history of the hunchback. Similarly, Quasimodo has transcended his 1831 (con)text in Victor Hugo's *Notre Dame de Paris*, not least in its re-titling in English as *The Hunchback of Notre Dame*, and continually revisits our screens in new incarnations (e.g., a new Hollywood production is in the works at the time of writing this chapter). Yet representations of hunchbacks go back thousands of years. In the United States, New York City's Metropolitan Museum of Art holds a piece dated from the twelfth to ninth century BCE, from the Olmec culture of Mexico (The Metropolitan Museum of Art, 2013). In her description of the piece, Associate Curator Heidi King observes that the 'social status and perception' of hunchbacks in early American societies is not known, but extrapolates from sixteenth-century Mexican and Peruvian records that 'misshapen persons' were 'held in awe', their difference associated with the possession of occult powers and considered good luck (King, 1990). She observes that Precolumbian hunchback figures are commonly found in burial sites (King, 1990). She notes that figurine is typical of Olmec work in its 'high degree of realism in posture and expression' and notes the particular attention given to 'the working of the facial features': this representation was realistic, not the synecdoche of impairment familiar to contemporary understanding of disability (King, 1990). The museum's *Heilbrunn Timeline of Art History* surmises that the figurine 'may have been a personal possession, perhaps belonging to a ruler or one who desired to keep the supernatural powers of a hunchback close at hand', and notes that later representations of hunchbacks 'depict them as members of royal courts, where they may have been due to the ruler's desire to commune with the supernatural realm to which the hunchbacks were thought to have access' (The Metropolitan Museum of Art, 2013). Indeed, hunchbacked figures recur in later Mesoamerican sculpture, across the Colima and Lagunillas cultures in the first to third centuries CE, up until the sixteenth century CE, when they were depicted on beakers and other water vessels by Peru's Inka and Chimú cultures.

Although there are many fragmentary appearances of hunchbacks across cultures after this, there is no room even to mention all these instances here. Furthermore, many of these appearances need much more primary research to reveal the full extent and context of their meaning in a truly useful way. Arguably the first prominent text to offer an opportunity for a fuller literary analysis is 'The Hunchback's Tale' from *The Arabian Nights*. This collection of Persian, Arabic, Indian, and Chinese folk and fairy tales, some of which can be traced back to the eighth century CE, was first aggregated into the form familiar to contemporary audiences in fifteenth century Egypt. The first two direct Arabic-to-English translations, by Torrens and Lane respectively, appeared in 1838, and had considerable influence on Western art, in particular the Romantics (Cecil, 1966).

Given its diverse origins and versions, 'The Hunchback's Tale' is particularly significant as an example of a disjuncture of meaning in cultural representations of the hunchback; it would be illuminating to conduct an in-depth comparison of the various versions of the text and trace shifts in meaning and the cultural attitudes associated with them. However, the provenance of these 'original' versions is problematic: 'the final compilation or redaction of the Hunchback Cycle' cannot be dated earlier than 1416, and so the overall structure of the manuscript may have affected the evolution of this individual story (Grotzfeld, 1991). Furthermore, although both Persian and Arabic elements have been identified (Abbott, 1949), other sources are as yet unidentified. Most significant of all is the observation that 'The Hunchback's Tale' contains '[o]ne of the most interesting and intricate developments – in terms of both the proliferation of narratives and the complex relationship between action and narrative' (Rosenthal, 1990: 120). The basic structure of the tale centres on the physical passing of the 'dead' hunchback's body, in 'slapstick fashion', among four men, each of whom believes that he has killed him (Rosenthal, 1990). The passing of the body thus drives the narrative, bridging each section and initiating the actions of a new focal character (Rosenthal, 1990: 120). When this sequence finally reaches its end, with the Sultan/King's remark 'Did ye ever hear a more wondrous tale than that of my Hunchback?', a new sequence begins, wherein the four men involved in handling the body seek to win a pardon by telling the most wondrous tale, a sequence that culminates in the tailor's story, which introduces the barber who discovers that the hunchback is not dead after all (Rosenthal, 1990: 120). Structurally, then, 'The Hunchback's Tale' fits David Mitchell and Sharon Snyder's concept of narrative prosthesis insofar as the impaired body is what makes the story possible. Simultaneously, we might note parallels for the way in which the general figure of the hunchback has been handled, and handed on, across cultures and through history.

Thinking about the hunchback

If narrative prosthesis has greater historical and cross-cultural reach than expected, it is also powerful enough to reach beyond literature itself. As mentioned, any attempt to document the history of representation of the figure of the hunchback must not limit itself to fiction, but also consider the way in which the hunchback identity of real people has shaped and been shaped by culture. In 'The Quasimodo complex' – which I first encountered in the collection *The Tyranny of the Normal* – Jonathan Sinclair Carey (then Director of the Institute of Ethics of Surgery) offers a physical and psychological diagnosis of the eponymous literary character, and then generalises that analysis to disabled people as a whole (Carey, 1996). As with the body in 'The Hunchback's Tale', the hunchback's body is passed between competing narratives, as both object and spur in the bizarre struggle between fiction and reality. For example, there is the argument that by 'all medical odds', Quasimodo 'should have been stillborn' (Carey, 1996: 34). This medical diagnosis of a literary character may seem absurd, but it simply illustrates the way in which fiction and reality meet in culture. The tussle between literary and medical narratives over disability has already been observed in relation to sideshows (Adams, 2001) and freakery (Garland-Thomson, 1996). In this context, we might, then, read Carey's words as an assertion of medicine's primacy over literature in the definition of a character. Yet literature resists: it is to Carey's regret that Quasimodo was not born 'severely retarded ... to keep him from awareness of his own lack of fleshly perfection' (Carey, 1996: 34).

At the same time, Carey awards literature more power than it actually has when he asserts that it 'records ... memorable scenes of self-perception about deformity' (Carey, 1996: 41). This may be true of some specific life-writing that we may classify as literature (e.g., Lucy Grealy's *Autobiography of a Face*, 2003), but Carey's attempt to apply this to literature in general reveals a certain naivety about literary texts. Beyond this, his main insights are that studies have shown that 'the deformed' have poor social skills, and that they 'may also hold an ... unexpressed fear of procreation' (Carey, 1996: 43). These are neither new, nor particularly insightful observations. The grand-sounding 'Quasimodo complex' is simply a restatement of a familiar idea: that the 'physically deformed' will be mentally maladjusted, or as Amy Lowell put it, 'Deformed body, deformed mind', which in itself would appear of a piece with the 'deformities of character' attributed to patients with physical deformities by Freud in 'The Exceptions' (cited in Garland-Thomson, 1996: 37). The lack of context for Carey's argument is apparent in his decision to conclude his case by quoting 'hunchbacked Englishman' William Hay on how the effects of deformity are 'intimately known to none but those who feel them; and they are generally inclined not to reveal them' (Carey, 1996). It should be pointed out that Hay was not simply a 'hunchbacked Englishman', but also a Member of Parliament, a role which is arguably of at least similar significance to the history of public life as that of writer (Nussbaum, 1997). Carey uses Hay's words to conclude, problematically, that literature reveals 'more about the sufferings of the deformed, with varying degrees of sympathy, than the deformed themselves do in direct discourse' (Carey, 1996: 46). Thus, fiction can trump reality once more – as in the case of Richard.

The attitudes toward disability apparent in histories by writers such as Skidmore are by no means adequate to act as buffers against the claims for fiction over reality offered by the likes of Carey (Longmore, 1985). If we are to deal with the figure of the hunchback specifically, rather than the broader political category of disability (which is problematic for the reasons described by Williams), Dante Germino's approach to Italian political theorist Antonio Gramsci might serve as an effective model. This approach begins with a characterisation of Gramsci's work as having 'a propensity to reunite philosophy and direct personal experience' (Germino, 1986: 20). Yet, 'how puzzling it is' to read analyses 'without finding a word about the impact of Gramsci's physical deformity on his life and thought', as his twisted spine 'had a far greater effect on his design for a new politics than did any reading he did':

That Antonio Gramsci was a gobbo (hunchback) helped make him enormously more attentive to the plight of individuals and groups 'at the margins of history'. The central theme of Gramsci's political theory was also the central preoccupation of his personal experience. For a long time, his hunchbacked condition made him feel like an 'intruder' in his own family, to say nothing of how he felt in relation to the 'fossilized' Sardinian attitudes that condemned and ridiculed any deviation from the norm (Germino, 1986: 21). Thus, Gramsci's central theme of the need for a new politics to focus on 'the world of the *emarginati* (those outside the margin of "respectable" society)' reflects two key aspects of his formative experiences 'as a doubly marginalized person', as hunchback and Sardinian (Germino, 1986: 21).

Gramsci was unaware that the medical condition Pott's disease caused his twisted spine, so he may 'have believed his mother's most unlikely story that his condition was the result of a fall down a flight of stairs' as a child (Germino, 1986: 21). This is an important point, in the light of the earlier material on the collision of fact and fiction in popular assumption, but not one that Germino explores further. Regardless of his conception of its cause, however, Germino firmly ascribes motivations to Gramsci's condition: 'his deformity had two effects: to make him feel like an outsider and to make him determined to transcend his handicap through contributing to humanity's advance' (Germino, 1986: 22). While this may appear to threaten to individualise his subject's experience, Germino insists that the emphasis on human will in Gramsci's work 'is almost certainly related to his own struggles to overcome his physical disadvantages' – in other words, his experience did contribute to a broader social movement on behalf of the marginalised and oppressed (Germino, 1986: 22). Problematically, however, Germino attributes this insight to an unnamed source who 'shared these feelings with me and ... stressed their importance for understanding Gramsci' (Germino, 1986: 29). Although this may appear worryingly similar in theme to Carey's reasoning, Germino's pursuit of this angle is redeemed by his focus on concrete links to Gramsci's drawing upon personal experience in his theoretical and political writing. Nevertheless, Germino is not immune to missing the broader context of a hunchback identity. At one point, he declares: 'There have been many hunchbacked people in history, but only Gramsci has produced a vision of politics worthy of study' (Germino, 1986: 22). As we have seen with thinkers such as Hay and Bourne, this is not necessarily true, even though Gramsci's influence on contemporary political thought has been more immediately apparent.

Nevertheless, Germino at least acknowledges the significance of Gramsci's curved spine in any complete picture of his work. He cites Gramsci's letters to his future wife Julia Schucht, which describe his family's attempts to cure his condition, through superstitious methods and makeshift harnesses (Germino, 1986). Gramsci also wrote of how hard it was to make friends as a child, and how he wore a 'mask of hardness' to 'conceal the despair he felt over his loneliness' (Germino, 1986: 23). Germino highlights the fact that Gramsci picked examples of disability to illustrate his political concern with those on the periphery: such as a teenager with learning disabilities chained up by his mother, and the woman who sought to drive her mother mad so that the state would institutionalise her (Germino, 1986: 23).

Some of Germino's observations of Gramsci's concerns are particularly pertinent to disability studies. For example, he shows how Gramsci was interested in the way in which radical protest was defined as 'pathological' (Germino, 1986). This use of medical authority to discredit difference is familiar to both disability studies scholars and disability rights activists. Similarly, Germino highlights Gramsci's belief that 'philanthropy' – the centre's voluntary sharing of some privilege with the periphery – will result only in further marginalisation: an idea that resonates with disability studies' critiques of charity (Germino, 1986: 23). More broadly, Gramsci's key contribution to political philosophy was the supplementation of Marx's idea of class struggle with his own experience of the exclusion practiced between the centre and the periphery. Gramsci's model thus 'makes room for the world of culture' (Germino, 1986: 24). In this regard, Gramsci's work offers a potential link between the political and cultural concerns of disability studies, and may be the best point of entry to the history of the hunchback from a contemporary perspective.

Conclusion

As mentioned at the start of this chapter, a proper analysis of the history of the cultural representation of the hunchback would require a book-length project. What is attempted here is a demonstration of the utility of focusing on a trans-historical figure to trace the development of attitudes toward disability. I demonstrate the power of those attitudes, in examples of fiction trumping fact, and show how a history of individuals and groups touched by disability lacks proper understanding without an appreciation of the context of their disability experience: for individuals marked as 'hunchbacks' therefore, this must take into account a history of representation and ascribed cultural meaning that spans thousands of years. History is, inevitably, textual, and so our living history is constructed, in part, on the attitudes and interpretations of historians and prominent commentators. In this regard, the hunchback has a usefully clear timeline: as curvatures of the spine are eliminated by medicine, so we must be careful not to lose the opportunity to document and understand the functioning of culture that this prominent unifying figure represents.

References

Abbott, N. (1949) A ninth-century fragment of the 'thousand nights': new light on the early history of the Arabian nights, *Journal of Near Eastern Studies*, 8, 3, 129–64.

Adams, R. (2001) *Sideshow U.S.A.: Freaks and the American Cultural Imagination*, Chicago: University of Chicago Press.

Bourne, R. (1911) The handicapped, *The Atlantic Monthly*, CV111, 320–29.

Carey, J.S. (1996) The Quasimodo complex, in C. Donley and S. Buckley (eds) *The Tyranny of the Normal: An Anthology*, Kent, Ohio: Kent State University Press.

Cecil, L.M. (1966) Poe's 'Arabesque', *Comparative Literature*, 18, 1, 55–70.

Fisher, M. (2013) Amazing photo of King Richard III's tiny, curved spine proves Shakespeare was wrong, *The Washington Post*, February 4, 2013.

Garland-Thomson, R. (1996) *Freakery: Cultural Spectacles of the Extraordinary Body*, New York: New York University Press.

Germino, D. (1986) Antonio Gramsci: From the margins to the center, the journey of a hunchback, *Boundary 2*, 14, 3, *The Legacy of Antonio Gramsci*, 19–30.

Grealy, L. (2003) *Autobiography of a Face*, London: Harper Perennial.

Grotzfeld, S. (1991) Book review. *The Arabian nights*, tr. by Husain Haddawy. New York: W.W. Norton, 1990, *Middle East Journal*, 45, 3, 519–20.

King, H. (1990) Recent acquisitions: a selection, 1989–1990, *The Metropolitan Museum of Art Bulletin*, 48, 2, 80.

Knight, S. and Lund, M.A. (2013) Richard Crookback, *The Times Literary Supplement*. Online. Available www.the-tls.co.uk/tls/public/article1208757.ece (accessed 1 September 2013)

Longmore, P. (1985) The life of Randolph Bourne and the need for a history of disabled people, *Reviews in American History* (December), 581–87.

Nussbaum, F.A. (1997) Feminotopias: the pleasures of 'deformity' in mid-eighteenth-century England, in D.T. Mitchell and S.L. Snyder (eds) *The Body and Physical Difference*, Ann Arbor: University of Michigan Press.

Rosenthal, M.M. (1990) Burton's literary Uroburos: 'The Arabian Nights' as self-reflexive narrative, *Pacific Coast Philology*, 25, 1/2, 116–25.

Skidmore, C. (2013) The hunchback is dead – long live Good King Richard, *The Daily Telegraph*. Online. Available www.le.ac.uk/richardiii/science/spine.html (accessed 29 October 2013).

The Metropolitan Museum of Art (2013) Hunchback [Mexico; Olmec] (1989.392) *Heilbrunn Timeline of Art History*. Online. Available www.metmuseum.org/toah/works-of-art/1989.392 (accessed 7 November 2013)

University of Leicester (2013) *Myths and Legends*. Online. Available www.le.ac.uk/richardiii/history/myths.html (accessed 29 October 2013).

Williams, K.S. (2009) Enabling Richard: the rhetoric of disability in Richard III, *Disability Studies Quarterly*, 29, 4.

7 Altered men

War, body trauma, and the origins of the cyborg soldier in American science fiction

Sue Smith

This chapter provides a preliminary inquiry into a strand of American science fiction literature that features the technological augmentation of the wounded hero – a man whose impaired/destroyed body is reconstructed into a human-machine. The significance of these works is that they emerge during moments of war and at times of new technological developments, often exploring the fantasy of the creation of enhanced human beings, while also reflecting anxieties about the impaired male body in relation to human and gender identity at the time of their publication. In order to explore the association of these texts within the broader historical events of war and within the social and cultural concerns of technology and the impaired and gendered body, I analyse two short stories. The first is Henry Kuttner's 'Camouflage' (first published in 1945), which I read in relation to the closing stages of World War II. The second is Joan D. Vinge's 'Tin Soldier' (first published in 1974), which I read in relation to the Vietnam War. The aim is to demonstrate how the work of male and female writers, writing within different historical contexts of war and gender politics, reflect changing cultural attitudes toward the wounded hero through shifting representations of the cyborg soldier.

The impaired/destroyed body and the rise of the human-machine

In American science fiction, speculation on the reconstruction of the impaired/ destroyed body into a human-machine emerged during the closing stages of World War II, coinciding with and anticipating advances in the development of prosthetics and a new science called cybernetics. Cybernetics incorporated theories about communication, engineering, and biology, establishing a scientific discourse that associated humans with machines (Hayles, 1999: 84). Of particular significance was the work of scientist Norbert Wiener, who calculated human-machine response times between pilots and their fighter planes in order to perfect anti-aircraft weaponry (Hayles, 1999: 86). Wiener's work suggested how technology could extend the capabilities of humans, giving scientific grounding to the concept of a human-machine relationship that we now commonly imagine as the cyborg figure.

The human-machine in cybernetics resonated with wartime images of modern prosthetics because, as David Serlin explains in 'The other arms race', it was a time when media images of disabled war veterans and 'the triumphant use of their prostheses' offered a positive fantasy of a human-machine relationship (Serlin, 2006: 52). At the same time, this popular image of the disabled war veteran was extremely problematic because the 'rehabilitation of amputees' was 'geared towards making able-bodied people more comfortable' with 'the disabled' (Serlin, 2006: 52). For example, rehabilitation programmes focused on encouraging individuals to use their prosthetics to regain a normal life. This meant that an amputee's goal was to achieve the human and gendered norms of western culture. I agree with Serlin's analysis of the disabled war veteran. Nonetheless, I also consider that the disabled war veteran as a human-machine fantasy helped shape a particular strand of cyborg literature in American science fiction. Utilising the concept of the rehabilitated impaired body, this literature often represented men as augmented beings, such as human-spaceships or human-weapons, expressing patriarchal desires about men as invincible and immortal human-machines, who could endure hostile environments and situations, pioneering new frontiers for the good of humanity, while also expressing society's fears about the human becoming subservient, even obsolete, in a new technological age.

Human-machine narratives provided meditations on what it might mean to be different in a world dominated by humans, offering insight into a cyborg's subjective experience of Otherness. At the same time, many writers revealed a gender bias in their work that favoured the superior status of the human male subject over the cyborg figure. Usually, this took the form of some kind of proof, or reassurance, that the human is central to the cyborg's existence, reasserting male authority and masculine control over the machine components that comprise the cyborg's identity. Examples that reflect this narrative formula begin in 1945 with Kuttner's 'Camouflage', and continue with classic science fiction literature such as Paul Anderson's short story 'Call me Joe' (first published in 1957), Robert Heinlein's military space opera *Starship Troopers* (first published in 1959), Martin Caiden's best-selling novel *Cyborg* (first published in 1972), and William Gibson's cyberpunk narratives of the 1980s, such as *Neuromancer* (first published in 1984), to name just a few. In addition to literature, the image of the reconstructed wounded hero has found expression in popular cinema such as in the *RoboCop Trilogy* (1987, 1990,1993) of the late 1980s and early 1990s and, more recently, in high profile mainstream films, such as James Cameron's *Avatar* (2009) and Duncan Jones's *Source Code* (2011). An enduring feature of these works is how they reaffirm human authority and masculine control over the technology that sustains the cyborg figure.

Often, in these narratives, the human is an elite, or respected member of society, usually a scientist, soldier, or astronaut, who is part of a covert military operation or a space expedition, and has been damaged and impaired in an accident or in a battle and reconstructed into a cyborg. Initially, as a being that is both organic and artificial, the cyborg questions the boundaries that separate humans from machines, rendering human identity problematic by highlighting that the human is a tentative and fragile construct. At the same time, the male protagonist is enabled by technology eliding his disability, as his human and masculine status is restored once more. Nonetheless, despite this resolution, a recurring anxiety evident in these texts is the way the reconstruction of the impaired/destroyed male body into a cyborg de-naturalises, questions, and exposes the constructed nature of human and gender identity in western culture. This is most evident in texts that emerge during times of great social upheaval such as war, when concerns about gender identity and gender roles are at their most sensitive. An example I now look at in order to explore these points further is Kuttner's 'Camouflage', an early narrative in American science fiction that provides the model for the many texts that were to follow.

World War II and Henry Kuttner's 'Camouflage'

'Camouflage' was originally published in *Astounding Science Fiction*, in September 1945, and is a story about an atomic scientist called Bart Quentin, whose body is destroyed in an accident, but whose brain is salvaged and re-housed in a 'two-foot-by-two-foot' metal cylinder so that it can easily be fitted into and used to control a ship that transports atomic power plants across space (Kuttner, 1961: 56). Despite his unusual human-machine guise, Kuttner has his protagonist go to great lengths to prove that he is still human and still a man, by demonstrating an ability to successfully assimilate technology into his life and also by outwitting a gang of criminals who try to hijack both his ship and his cargo for their own ends. Primarily, Quentin's humanness is tested by a character called Van Talman, who is a former acquaintance of his, and a gang member. When Talman first meets Quentin, he is unsettled by his human-machine identity. However, Quentin is quick to emphasise how his ability to pilot a ship is enhanced through his 'synthesis with a machine': 'Ever noticed, when you're driving or piloting, how you identify with the machine? It's an extension of you. I go one step farther. And it's satisfying' (Kuttner, 1961: 58). Quentin even goes on to declare, 'I am the machine!' but is careful to emphasise that he is no robot: 'It doesn't affect my identity, the personal essence of Bart Quentin' (Kuttner, 1961: 58).

In Kuttner's narrative, being human is defined through a vague and unquantifiable category, 'personal essence', and his masculinity is demonstrated by his 'natural' ability to exercise his dominance over machinery that he relies on for sustaining his social and economic existence. This allows Quentin to occupy a social function acceptable and amenable to patriarchal values that constitute male identity. In this respect, Quentin's socially defined gender, already established in the narrative in his role as a scientist, is reaffirmed through an occupation conventionally befitting a man. He is a pilot and controller of a space ship, allowing his masculine identity to be re-mapped seamlessly onto his biological identity, his brain. In other words, despite Quentin's lack of an organic body, the narrative allows Quentin's unusual form and difference to be accommodated, promoting him as a new kind of human fit for space travel.

Quentin's ability to supersede the limitations of his physical body without compromising his masculine identity and his humanness is further proved by his intellectual capacity finally to outwit his hijackers. In a final showdown with his assailants, Quentin kills all but one of the criminals, his former friend, Talman. Talman attempts to out-manoeuvre Quentin by engaging him in a conversation that is meant to psychologically undermine his self-worth and value as both a man and a human. However, as Anne Hudson Jones explains, in her article 'The Cyborg (R)evolution in Science Fiction', just as Quentin starts to doubt his own status, 'Only a semantic slip restores his sense of himself as human' (Jones, 1982: 206). In a lapse of concentration, Talman claims that he would never have tried to kill Quentin, if Quentin were still human. At this point Quentin realises Talman's mistake, because as he points out, 'A machine can be stopped or destroyed Van ... But it can't be – *killed*' (Kuttner, 1961: 84). Knowing that Quentin is 'still perceived as human is sufficient to restore Quentin's sense of himself as human' (Jones, 1982: 206).

Although Kuttner's narrative does not directly refer to war, and Quentin is not explicitly a cyborg soldier, the title 'Camouflage' implicitly carries military connotations, reflecting the tactics used by our male protagonist, who emerges as an efficient killing machine in order to defend his environment, his ship, and its valuable resources. Furthermore, the timing of Kuttner's publication and the subject matter that details the personal journey of a man who has experienced severe body trauma and, with the aid of technology, endeavours to regain his human and masculine identity, resonates with the war-time media images of disabled war veterans and their 'triumphant use of prostheses' (Serlin, 2006: 52). I would argue that the treatment of Bart Quentin's character by Kuttner in fact resonates with broader social issues that emerged in the closing years of World War II, such as concerns about returning war veterans, particularly disabled war veterans and their rehabilitation into civilian life, and the re-establishment of the gendered social order for a post-war era. As a consequence of these concerns, an extensive social programme in countries such as North America was developed to reinstate the war veteran. This included designing and promoting prosthetics along the lines of socially sanctioned, gendered roles, which reconstructed and normalised the individual as 'naturally' masculine. For example, in 'Engineering Masculinity: Veterans and Prosthetics after World War Two', Serlin discusses an image of a man with a prosthetic arm lighting a cigarette:

> Professional photographs of veteran amputees using new prosthetic devices to perform "normal" male activities – such as lighting and enjoying a cigarette – were deliberate attempts to challenge the reputation of the male amputee as ineffectual and effeminate.
>
> (Serlin, 2002: 61)

Serlin makes it clear that although the reality of life for returning veterans with amputations was a far cry from the propaganda images of military and state funded social programs, the preference nevertheless was to rehabilitate impaired male bodies 'to assume the idealized stature of "real" American men' (Serlin, 2002: 46).

Similarly, the reconstruction of gender 'norms' through the rehabilitation of the impaired/destroyed body is central to Kuttner's science fiction narrative. In

Kuttner's story, Bart Quentin's new identity as a human machine is fully accommodated, not only by the satisfactory resolution of a story that reinstates Quentin's human and masculine status by having him engage in combat and defeat his foe, but also by the presence of a loyal, adoring wife, Linda, who acknowledges his dominance and authority over her. Despite the fact that her husband resides in a two-foot-by-two cylinder, Linda is able to adjust to his new if unusual physical status as a human-machine. For example, when Linda Quentin directly addresses Bart's former friend Van Talman, she insists, 'He's still Bart,' […] 'He may not look it, but he's the man I married alright' (Kuttner, 1961: 56). The faithful and unfailingly loyal wife or girlfriend was a recurring motif in the post war years, because, as Rebecca Jo Plant points out in 'The Veteran, his Wife and their Mothers: Prescriptions for Psychological Rehabilitation after World War II', 'experts pressured young women to resume traditional feminine roles, placing their husbands' needs above their own' (Plant, 1999: 2). The same was true for those women whose returning husbands or sweethearts were physically disabled veterans (Plant, 1999: 2). This social attitude toward women's role in the rehabilitation and acceptance of the returning wounded hero is exemplified in Kuttner's tale.

To sum up at this point, we might argue that Kuttner's short story is an early example of cyborg fiction that resonates with issues concerning war, body trauma and anxieties about disability and gender at the time of its publication. The reconstruction of the impaired/destroyed body through advanced technology and the reinstatement of the human and gender identity of the wounded male hero, in accordance with the preferred gendered social order in patriarchal culture, are key motifs. Therefore it is crucial that the narrative ensures the male protagonist prove his humanness, which, ultimately, is at the centre of the cyborg's identity, as well as his masculinity (and heterosexuality), which is reaffirmed by a love interest, such as a loyal girlfriend or wife. Furthermore, it is a narrative formula that has often been repeated in science fiction culture, reassuring anxieties about impairment and the limitations of the human body, eliding any disturbing images of disability. However, I now look at a text by a woman whose 'Tin Soldier', originally published in Damon Knight's anthology *Orbit 14*, draws upon and emphasises anxieties that the figure of the wounded hero generates in patriarchal culture. I argue that Vinge's short story critiques the image of the invincible cyborg soldier in science fiction and the macho culture of war.

The Vietnam war veteran and Joan D. Vinge's 'Tin Soldier'

'Tin Soldier' is about a man called Maris, who is injured in combat and reconstructed into a cyborg. Rejecting war he travels to another planet where he falls in love with a woman space traveller called Brandy. In his new environment, Maris realises that, as a cyborg existing outside of his warring culture, he is marginalised by society: 'He wakened' in a place where there were, 'no wars and almost no people. And found out that now to the rest of humanity he was no longer quite human' (Vinge, 1976: 245). Maris's marginal status in a world dominated by humans is emphasised through the careful juxtaposing of organic and artificial parts that constitute his human-machine identity:

> His face was ordinary, with eyes that were dark and patient, and his hair was coppery barbed wire bound with a knotted cloth. Under the curling copper, under the skin, the back of his skull was a plastic plate. The quick fingers of the hand ... were plastic, the smooth arm was prosthetic.
>
> (Vinge, 1976: 200)

Maris's high-tech body is viewed as strange and frightening, he is a marginal figure, but his status as a cyborg is tolerated, and he is allowed to own and run a bar called Tin Soldier, which is frequented by female space travellers. One night he meets Brandy and falls in love with her. Brandy breaks the ultimate taboo by engaging in a sexual liaison with a cyborg. Finally, she falls in love with Maris.

In 'Tin Soldier', the male cyborg does not try to prove his humanness nor does he embark on a personal quest to regain his masculinity, but rather the presence of his human-machine identity questions the warring macho culture that has marginalised him. 'Tin Soldier' is a feminist anti-war text that is oppositional to conventional representations of the male cyborg in science fiction. Vinge's cyborg draws directly from the problematic image of the disabled Vietnam War veteran that emerged in American culture during the 1970s. When Vinge's short story was first published in 1974, the term *tin soldier* held a prominent place in North America's conscience. 'One Tin Soldier' was an anti-war song that became popular with students and the counter-culture scene. Testifying to its popularity, 'One Tin Soldier' was named 'Number One All Time Requested Song of 1971 and 1973 by the American Radio Broadcasters Association' (Songfacts, 2009: 1; Punish, 2010: 4).

'One Tin Soldier' is a song that rejects violence, but by the time the Vietnam War was over and the veterans returned home, the song also came to represent a rejection of those who took part in the conflict. Returning veterans, particularly those disabled by the war, did not come home to a hero's welcome, but were instead treated as social pariahs. In 'Bitterness, Rage and Redemption: Hollywood Constructs the Disabled Vietnam Veteran', Martin F. Norden argues that in American culture, filmmakers rewrote history and placed the blame for the Vietnam War 'on a few self-destructive and "Otherized" soldiers – to make them bear ... "the stigma of guilt for the whole society"' (Norden, 2003: 108). Unlike the disabled veterans of World War II, who were portrayed as having earned their citizenship through their commitment and self-sacrifice, the disabled Vietnam War veteran's rehabilitation into society was less straightforward. The Vietnam conflict was unpopular and, furthermore, was perceived to be an un-winnable war that blighted America's liberal ideals and military history. While there was a concerted effort to restore the masculine status of the disabled veteran of World War II (because he was deemed worthy), the disabled Vietnam War veteran was considered a problematic figure.

In Vinge's 'Tin Soldier', Maris is also an Othered War Veteran. He knows that his status as a cyborg not only makes him subordinate to women, but also positions him outside the world of men. At times he recalls bitterly the moment he sustained his injuries in war:

> And the memory filled him of how it felt to be nineteen, and hating war, and blown to pieces ... to find yourself suddenly half-prosthetic, with the pieces that were gone still hurting in your mind; and your stepfather's voice, with something that was not pride, saying you were finally a real man [...].
>
> (Vinge, 1976: 244–45)

Maris's words are ironic. He has not returned from war as a 'real man' but has become something else, which a war veteran of another generation cannot understand. Vinge's male protagonist reflects the alienation and discrimination that disabled Vietnam veterans faced in civilian life during the 1970s. He is a soldier who has survived because of advances made in technology and medicine, but he also possesses an identity that creates a sense of unease in those around him. The most disturbing aspect of Maris's identity is the liminality of his body. Maris is a cyborg and is considered to be no longer a living man. It is only technology that animates what is left of his organic body. When Brandy informs Maris that she has discussed their night together with the other spacer women, Maris assures her that her action will not overcome their xenophobia. As Maris states, 'to most people in most cultures cyborgs are unnatural, the next thing up from a corpse' (Vinge, 1976: 205). To the spacer women, Brandy's transgression is a perversion – as Maris explains, to sleep with a cyborg, 'You'd have to be a necrophile' (Vinge, 1976: 205). In contrast to Kuttner's narrative, where the body of the wounded hero is concealed and hidden from view, the body of the cyborg in 'Tin Soldier' is visible and open to the gaze of others who fear the vulnerability and mortality that it signifies.

Vinge's and Kuttner's texts are from different moments in twentieth-century history and reflect the gender politics of their time. In Kuttner's 'Camouflage', the narrative reflects the desire to return the wounded hero to a gendered social order ready for a new post-war era. In Vinge's 'Tin Soldier' the gendered social order, underpinned by a culture of violence and war, is questioned, utilising the image of the wounded hero to promote a utopian feminist future. For example, in the final pages of the story, Brandy is damaged in a fire and becomes a cyborg like Maris. Brandy mourns the loss of her privileged life as a spacer woman and the freedom this life offered her, but she also asks Maris 'How do you bear it?' to which he replies, 'By learning what really matters ... Worlds are not so small. We'll go to other worlds if you want – we could see Home ... And maybe in time the rules will change' (Vinge, 1976: 247). It is not Brandy who offers the final words of hope. Instead, the hope of an alternative future beyond patriarchy comes from Maris, the physically impaired war veteran. Maris rejects the warring culture that has made him into who he is and embraces a future that maintains him in a marginal position – it is a future shared by a man and a woman who love and respect each other on equal terms. Overall, in her promotion of a utopian future, Vinge looks beyond the human and utilises the cyborg as a figure of hope for social transformation and gender equality.

Conclusion

In this chapter I introduce and discuss Kuttner's 'Camouflage', which marks the beginning of a strand of cyborg narratives in American science fiction that speculate on the possibility of interfacing technology with the body of the wounded hero. I discuss the significance of this text in relation to issues such as war, body trauma, disability, and gender at the time of its publication, arguing that it is a text that resonates with concerns about the rehabilitation of the disabled war veteran at the end of World War II. I also provide a comparative reading of a cyborg text by a woman science fiction writer in order to highlight how male and female writers in different social contexts create work that reflect shifting attitudes toward gender and disability through the image of the disabled war veteran. The chapter only allows me to touch on a fraction of what can be said about the representation of the wounded hero in American science fiction, and is far from complete in its survey. The aim is to develop this work further and to contribute to disability studies scholarship by offering a broader and more comprehensive account of society's fascination with the cyborg, commonly represented through the impaired/destroyed body reconstructed into a human-machine.

References

Anderson, P. (1973) Call me Joe, in B. Bova (ed.) *The Science Fiction Hall of Fame*, Volume Two A, New York: Double Day.

Avatar (2009) Film. Directed by James Cameron. [DVD] UK: Twentieth Century Fox.

Caiden, M. (1974) *Cyborg*, London: Mayflower.

Gibson, W. (1995) *Neuromancer*, London: HarperCollins.

Hayles, K.N. (1999) *How We Became Posthuman: Virtual Bodies in Cybernetics, Literature, and Informatics*, Chicago: University of Chicago Press.

Heinlein, R.A. (1982) *Starship Troopers*, London: New English Library.

Jones, A.H. (1982) The cyborg (r)evolution in science fiction, in T.P. Dunn and R.D. Erlich (eds) *The Mechanical God: Machines in Science Fiction*, Westport: Greenwood Press.

Kuttner, H. (1961) Camouflage, in H. Kuttner, *Ahead of Time*, London: Four Square.

Norden, M.F. (2003) Bitterness, rage and redemption: Hollywood constructs the disabled Vietnam veteran, in D.A. Gerber (ed.) *Disabled Veterans in History*, Ann Arbor: University of Michigan Press.

Plant, R.J. (1999) *The Veteran, His Wife And Their Mothers: Prescriptions For Psychological Rehabilitation After World War II*. 1999. Online. Available http://historyweb.ucsd.edu/pages/people/faculty%20pages/RPlantVeteransFinal.pdf 1-11. (accessed 16 September 2007).

Punish, J. (2010) *Billy Jack's 'One Tin Soldier' Gets Makeover for 2011: MarcyElle Belts out One Tin Soldier' for a New Generation*. Online. Available http://johnnypunish.com/blog/2010/12/billy-jack-one-tin-soldier/ 1–6. (accessed 20 October 2013).

RoboCop (1987) Film. Directed by Paul Verhoeven. [DVD] UK: Orion Pictures.

RoboCop 2 (1990) Film. Directed by Irvin Kershner. [DVD] UK: Orion Pictures.

RoboCop 3 (1993) Film. Directed by Fred Dekker. [DVD] UK: Orion Pictures.

Serlin, D. (2002) Engineering masculinity: veterans and prosthetics after World War Two, in K. Ott, D. Serlin, and S. Mihm (eds) *Artificial Parts, Practical Lives: Modern Histories of Prosthetics*, New York: New York University Press.

Serlin, D. (2006) The other arms race, in L.J. Davis (ed.) *The Disability Studies Reader*, New York: Routledge.

Songfacts. *One Tin Soldier (The Legend of Billy Jack) by Coven*. Online. Available www. songfacts.com/detail.php?id=3888. 1-6 (accessed 16 September 2009).

Source Code (2011) Film. Directed by Duncan Jones. [DVD] UK: Vendome Pictures.

Vinge, J.D. (1976) Tin Soldier, in P. Sargent (ed.) *More Women of Wonder*, London: Penguin.

8 The cultural work of disability and illness memoirs

Schizophrenia as collaborative life narrative

Stella Bolaki

Despite a hundred and more years' research since Emil Kraepelin's description in his *Clinical Psychiatry* of schizophrenia (or 'dementia praecox', as he called it), schizophrenia's neuropathology remains obscure. Angela Woods views schizophrenia as the 'sublime object' of psychiatry, that is, as its disciplinary limit point (Woods, 2011). Even though there are many competing theories, the condition is often described as a mental disorder occurring in people with a genetic vulnerability activated by psychosocial stressors. Outside clinical contexts, on the one hand, schizophrenia has been celebrated as an experience of the sublime, the transcendent, the liberating and the revolutionary in so called antipsychiatric models of schizophrenia coming out of various countercultural movements in Europe and America (Laing, 1965; Szasz, 1972; Deleuze and Guattari, 2009). On the other hand, it has been further pathologised by theorists such as Fredric Jameson and Jean Baudrillard who have turned it into the representative form of *postmodern* subjectivity.

Both models have been dismissed by many as being insensitive and inappropriate in that they use schizophrenia as a trope, metaphor, or symbol. Moreover, as often observed, such understandings of schizophrenia have been based on a few exceptional schizophrenics, most notably Judge Daniel Paul Schreber's *Memoirs of My Nervous Illness* (1903), commented on by the likes of Freud, Jung, Lacan, and Deleuze and Guattari. Contemporary personal accounts of schizophrenia should be placed in the context of a growing body of life narratives and of the rise more specifically of disability and illness narratives (across different media and circulating in various circles). These are produced by people who 'mark themselves specifically as non-exceptional [ordinary] schizophrenics' (Prendergast, 2008: 55) and claim the right to own their experiences by speaking publicly on those issues that affect their lives, including diagnosis, treatment, and stigma. The confessional impulse is a first step toward 'rhetorical ownership' and 'civic rhetoric' (Prendergast, 2008: 57, 60), and frequent criticisms that memoirs are individualistic, sentimental, or voyeuristic notwithstanding, it is hard to deny that one of the attractions of the form is its inclusive and democratic potential.

Despite the backlash against the contemporary memoir boom, many literary critics recognise that the genre can have 'strong ethical impulses' and 'powerful real-world effects' (Couser, 2012: 175). In this chapter I address on-going debates about schizophrenia and the kind of 'work' – social, cultural, and political – that contemporary narratives of illness and disability are capable of doing by focusing on *Henry's Demons: Living with Schizophrenia, A Father and Son's Story* (2011), co-written by Patrick and Henry Cockburn. The questions that frame my discussion of this memoir are a variation on those raised by Lisa Diedrich in her study *Treatments* in relation to a different set of contemporary illness narratives:

> What is it about the writing and reading of memoir that is potentially transformative? What sort of *knowledges* are articulated in [illness narratives]? How are those *knowledges* different from expert medical knowledges, and are they capable of transforming expert medical knowledges [and social attitudes about disability and illness]?
>
> (Diedrich, 2007)

Finally, and this is particularly pertinent to collaborative narratives, 'what sort of ethics emerges' out of writing and reading such narratives? (Diedrich, 2007: viii).

Henry's Demons as collaborative life narrative

Henry's Demons consists of chapters by Patrick and Henry (written from a first-person perspective) that alternate – one reviewer has described the effect as 'a duet' (Strauss, 2011). The experiment started with an article that the father and son published in a supplement of *The Independent* in September 2008 and later, encouraged by the positive reception it had, expanded into a book. In the memoir, the words *Patrick* and *Henry* serve as titles of individual chapters. Patrick's chapters, written from his 'outside' reporter perspective, are more journalistic or detached, in line with his professional style of writing (he is a war correspondent). As one reviewer notes, 'it is no exaggeration to say that the job of writing about his son Henry's descent into madness [was] the toughest assignment of Cockburn's career' (Linklater, 2011). This appears to be true given Patrick's admission in the book that 'the word "schizophrenia" did not mean very much to me, since I knew almost nothing about the illness except that it did not mean having a split personality' (Cockburn & Cockburn, 2011: 19). Here it is worth noting that Patrick engages with medical models from 'below' in the memoir – that is, not as an expert in mental health – thus offering an important and often critical perspective upon these forms of knowledge. This also differentiates the memoir from other co-authored books on schizophrenia commissioned with a more explicitly educational purpose such as *Me, Myself and Them* (Snyder et al., 2007).

Relational and collaborative life narratives have been recently embraced within auto/biography studies for challenging the myth of the autonomous self and transcending fixed generic boundaries (Miller, 1996; Eakin, 1999; Egan, 1999). From philosophical, ethical, and pedagogical perspectives, collaborative illness narratives explore and explode the opposition between health and illness; force us to confront the often disavowed realities of disability, aging, and death; and can be used to foster new practices of witnessing and caring for others. Despite these benefits, life writing critics have also drawn attention to the ethical dilemmas built into such narratives. In his appropriately entitled essay 'Making, Taking and Faking Lives: The Ethics of Collaborative Life Writing', Thomas Couser singles out 'the political imbalance latent in narratives of illness and disability ... most problematic in those cases in which the completion and publication of the narrative devolve upon a survivor who narrates another's terminal illness' (Couser, 1998: 334). Whose story is the final one and where does one draw the line between facilitating and appropriating the expression of another person's painful experience? Patrick explains in the Preface of the book that he did not wish to write another one of those 'best-selling but ghostwritten memoirs of so many sportsmen, generals, and politicians' and that 'Henry's firsthand testimony alone could convey what it is like to hear voices and see visions' (xiv). Still, Patrick has full editorial control: he writes most of the chapters (he is also the sole author of the Preface and the acknowledgements) and provides the overall framework for the book's structure, guiding his son's writing, as he has acknowledged in interviews and book readings.

Even though Patrick confesses in the Preface his worry about subjecting Henry to extra stress – unlike other memoirs written after the subject has recovered, Henry is 'well enough to write but not too distant from his psychosis' (xiv) – Patrick defends the project on other grounds: 'If, instead of telling people he was in a mental hospital, [Henry] could say he was writing a book about his experiences, it would be good for his morale and self-confidence' (212). In other words, Henry could dispel the myth that so-called mentally ill people are not productive members of society or are incapable of work. In addition, the book could serve 'a broader public purpose by making mental illness less of a mystery people are embarrassed to discuss' (xiii). This is of course not the first book with such a purpose, but Patrick finds it astonishing, as he works on the project, to discover that so many people he knows turn out to have a close family member who have the condition but feel inhibited to talk. A report from November 2012 by the independent Schizophrenia Commission entitled 'The Abandoned Illness' confirms that '87% of service users report experiences of stigma and discrimination'. When it comes to Henry's motivation for embarking on the project, it is not as clear but he gives his consent (and the doctors agree that Henry is well enough to write). As Patrick explains, 'it took a lot of coaxing and encouragement to get [Henry] to write' (xv) – which suggests some resistance on his part – but 'working on the book appeared to give him a sense of purpose and accomplishment' (212).

Rather than obliterating the voice and experience of the person represented (which may happen when the nature of the collaboration is not precise), clear boundaries are maintained between the father and son's voices throughout *Henry's Demons*. The alternation of chapters, especially the fact that the same episodes are revisited from Patrick's and Henry's perspectives, subtly allude to a process of weighing conflicting claims of perpetrators and victims during war times or while writing a news story. However, the book does not take sides when it comes to the events it presents, but illuminates both Henry's and Patrick's predicament through its bifocal view. One reviewer picks on this aspect of the collaborative narrative:

To his family, Henry's getaways – he escaped 30 times by his own account and several occasions almost died, once sitting naked under a tree in the snow for two days – seem fits of selfishness, which they are. How can he put his parents through these constant trials (readers may ask) if he knows he won't make it outside for long without cash, medicine, warm clothes? But to Henry who was sectioned in early 2003 and spent most of the following seven years in mental hospitals, they seem necessary, which they probably are, too: 'I felt a call from the natural world to run away from where I was incarcerated.'

(Strauss, 2011)

This double perspective is facilitated by the alternation of chapters and the overall narrative structure, but it does not only add to the dramatic effect of the memoir (the conflict between Henry and his family, typical of family memoirs that do not necessarily address illness). It also sustains a dialogue about understandings of mental illness. For example, even though Patrick mentions his hope that writing would be a way for Henry 'to admit that he had an illness' and start taking his medication (211), the Preface makes it clear that there is tension right from the onset of the project, a tension that, I argue, is productive: 'I [Patrick] run my idea for the book past [Henry] and he liked it though when we spoke of the hallucinations, he objected to the word, since to him they remain genuine events' (xiv). Thus, '*our* story of living with schizophrenia', which is how Patrick describes in the Preface the chapters that follow (xv, emphasis added), may point to a shared narrative between father and son, but the experiences that compose it are not identical.

The aesthetic and ethical work of illness narratives

With few exceptions, Western psychiatry acknowledges delusions as 'a principle symptom of schizophrenia', but reduces them to 'mere reflections, unimportant in their own right, of mechanisms determined by biological substrates' (Lovell, 1997: 456). Similarly, when it comes to auditory hallucinations, 'psychiatrists are only interested in certain very restricted features of the voices', such as whether the voices speak the patient's thoughts aloud or talk about the patient in the third person, so as to make their diagnosis of schizophrenia (Thomas, 1997: 19). Once a diagnosis is made, interpretation closes down. From a narrative and phenomenological perspective, however, accounts by people who have schizophrenia, including their interpretations of visual and auditory hallucinations or delusional language, represent a person's active attempts to make sense of her or his lived experiences in a way that is personally meaningful but can also be grasped by others. In this sense, illness narratives do not only serve a therapeutic purpose but have important ethical and social repercussions.

Recent work on illness narratives has underlined the importance of taking seriously 'the semantic and aesthetic potential' (Radley, 2009: 17) of such personal accounts, which is not synonymous with aestheticisation. For example, Alan Radley advocates 'a different way of talking about illness, a way that acknowledges that the representation of illness or suffering involves world-making, not just acts of interpretation and social judgement' (Radley, 2009: 42). This is perhaps more urgent for a condition like schizophrenia that has long been construed as a state of cognitive and affective deficit. Henry's chapters do not preclude agency, resistance, and emotional complexity. An example is the story Henry repeats in one of the chapters told to him by a nurse at the Priory hospital. Claren tells him that Australian aborigines put stones in their mouths so they produce saliva and have to drink less under the hot sun. Henry's response is revealing: 'I thought that Claren's story *related to me but in a different way*. I recalled that birds have no teeth and swallow stones to digest, so I thought that if I swallowed a stone, I would turn into a bird and be able to fly away from the Priory and all my troubles' (41, emphasis added). Rather than being a symptom of his exclusion from the 'real' world or a textual puzzle to be deciphered like a dream by the analyst, this story is a 'fragment' (Radley, 2009: 184–85) of a different world that Henry constructs and into which we are ushered as readers by bearing witness to it.

When considering Henry's delusional language and 'extravagant' requests, once again we see a communicating subject actively integrating past and present experiences, even though schizophrenia has been viewed in terms of being 'stuck' in time (Jameson, 1991). For example, when Henry asks his mother Jan to sing him a hymn in the hospital, it is not any hymn as Henry requests 'the hymn that you sang when we were coming back from Ireland', during a 'long, boring drive' (14). Jan, whose diary entries constitute one of the chapters, thus providing a third perspective, writes:

> [Henry] is not exactly talkative with Patrick and me, but not silent, either. He gets hold of a waste bin, turns it upside down, and plays it as a drum, improvising rhymed 'raps' as he's done before at bad times. 'O do de do, through the hawthorn the chill wind blows' – much like that. He seems almost oblivious of us all as he chants. (154)

However, we know, from previous mentions in the text (and here the father's and mother's account helps as it provides the broader context of Henry's life with his family) that the raps Henry tends to invent draw on past experiences: 'Through and through and on to Peru/ Through every taboo and on to Peru,' Henry raps in one of the chapters. Anticipating a response according to which schizophrenic language is no more than a senseless collection of syllables and neologisms, Henry adds, 'I had been in Peru for my cousin's wedding the year before' (33). Other raps are directly related to his experience of being legally restrained – one rap song he repeats to himself while expecting to be sectioned includes the word *section* (89) and another speaks of 'boredom and rage in a cage' (218). These songs seem to take the pain and other emotions associated with his experiences and translate it into something else. This is what Radley calls the 'work of illness' where aesthetic activity becomes a kind of 'work' and illness narratives can be understood as deriving their significance from 'the deployment of an ethic of freedom [for the person who is ill], realised in terms of aesthetic practice' (Radley, 2009: 38).

A final example is worth mentioning here: Patrick draws attention to Henry's 'worst breakdowns and brainstorms which [Henry] later nicknamed his "polka-dot days" though the phrase does not quite convey the terrors which then seemed to possess him' (158). This is precisely the purpose of such 'work' behind illness stories; writing about your experience creates 'a screen' through which the terrors of illness can be contemplated with distance by both author and readers (Radley, 2009: 184). Taking seriously the aesthetic dimension and imaginative work underlying illness narratives (and what better example than the translation of torments into 'polka dot days') is fundamental to the communication of illness, to both the one who has an illness and others who do not have access to it.

Transforming medical knowledges and social attitudes toward schizophrenia

But how does the book negotiate the actual question of diagnosis that is extremely powerful in shaping people's experience of so-called mental health problems and, it should be added, carries certain legal measures? Henry was sectioned, that is detained under section 3 of the Mental Health Act, for refusing to take his medication and being judged a risk to himself. 'Do I have schizophrenia?' he asks in one of the early chapters. 'I don't know. My mother, father and the dreaded psychiatrist definitely believe I am schizophrenic. They have grounds for their belief, such as my being found naked and talking to trees in the woods. Yet, I think I just see the world differently from other people, and maybe if psychiatrists understood this I wouldn't be in hospital' (43). As noted, Henry objects to the term *hallucination* and refers to what he sees as 'visions' (38). 'I am still not sure I am mentally ill', Henry writes toward the end of the memoir (221). Regarding what are clinically termed 'auditory hallucinations', Henry notes in neutral language, 'It is certain that I do hear voices and that some people do not hear voices' (221). He does not write for example that 'sane people' do not hear voices and when he adds that 'I remember when I didn't [hear voices]' (221) he indicates that this former state has changed but he does not pass any judgement on it. His comment has a normalising function in that it regards the experience of hearing voices as one of a wide range of possible forms of human experience. This also underlies the work of the Hearing Voices Network, established in Britain in 1990, which operates nationally and internationally in alliance with sympathetic professionals. This network, like other organisations and smaller groups, validates voice hearers' own accounts of their experiences and makes it possible for these experiences to become meaningful.

Henry refuses to take his medication on many occasions throughout the book because, as his mother puts it, 'he is defending his whole identity and integrity, and taking the drugs means that everything he thinks is wrong' (25). When his father tries to persuade him to take olanzapine by suggesting that it is 'the equivalent of the polio vaccine', Henry replies 'but you were really ill, and I am not', which makes Patrick hesitant to pursue a simplistic comparison between physical and mental illness (25). Henry's refusal to take antipsychotic drugs should not be dismissed as a form of denial. It is a personal strategy of protecting his sense of identity, but also has implications for how we understand the category of schizophrenia, particularly at a time when the successes of psychopharmacology have paved the way for predominantly biological theories (especially in the United States) and have put the priority on efficient technologies of treatment rather than more holistic approaches that take into consideration cultural factors. In his chapters, Patrick draws attention to studies that have revealed how migrant communities in different parts of the world are more susceptible to schizophrenia, which belies the idea of a solely biological origin behind this condition. Even though Henry's father does not doubt his son's membership within the category of the mentally ill person, he presents research that confirms that distinctions between different mental disorders, such as schizophrenia and bipolar disorder, are 'artificial' (100), and he reminds us that diagnosis in the United States and the United Kingdom does not follow exactly the same criteria (in terms of how early someone is diagnosed, for example). Very few people would contest the extraordinary diversity of the disorder, and with the publication of the fifth edition of the American Psychiatric Association's Diagnostic and Statistical Manual of Mental Disorders (DSM 5) in May 2013 and the eleventh revision of the World Health Organisation's International Classification of Diseases in 2014 these debates are likely to continue.

Outside the medical context, and especially in artistic circles, the label *schizophrenia* is applied loosely and even has positive associations as becomes apparent in Henry's opening chapter: 'The first time I heard the word "schizophrenic" was in an arts class ... Somebody had done a series of good drawings. The teacher said they "looked like the paintings of a schizophrenic"' (31). The link between creativity and madness or psychosis has been a long-term subject of research and debate and it is invoked on several occasions by both Patrick and Henry (references are made to Virginia Woolf and Jackson Pollock, for instance). Both Patrick and Henry draw to a certain extent on such understandings of schizophrenia as positive strategies that resist medical and pathologising discourses. Patrick describes Henry's artistic sensibility, and the book contains several sketches he drew before and after his diagnosis. Henry often calls his illness a 'spiritual awakening', a state giving access 'to another side to the world [he] hadn't seen before' (31), also reflected in some of the sketches. Patrick's research into what doctors call family history of mental illness in one of the chapters is equally interesting. One story Patrick offers is that of Hugh Montefiore's (Jan's father) 'spectacular and unexpected conversion to Christianity' that involved visions and voices. This happened in 1936 when he was sixteen. Patrick writes: 'His experience highlighted for me that it was possible to have some of the symptoms of schizophrenia without being mad or being seen as suffering from madness' (111).

While Patrick is suspicious about the connection between intelligence or originality and schizophrenia, he finds it more than 'a mechanism of emotional compensation for families who discovered that they were susceptible to the disease' (110). Approaching schizophrenic voices as no different from traditional religious or spiritual beliefs, however irrational to a doctor, can help a patient put one's experiences 'in a more manageable context', as shown by the story of Mark's recovery from schizophrenia told by Patrick in the book (107). Mark spent time with monks and people who 'took the idea of spiritual visions seriously as a path towards self-knowledge and did not see them in purely medical terms' (108). As Patrick notes, 'this was never going to happen at any of the hospitals Henry was in' (108). As mentioned before, the problem with most approaches to hallucinations, including cognitive behavioural therapy that does not negate their existence, is that the content and meaning of the voices are not important since the goal is to challenge subjects' beliefs about their voices, improve coping mechanisms, and reduce distress or even voice activity. Even though this is beneficial, it offers little help to those who want to understand the significance of their voices rather than defer to the expert's opinion. Spirituality and religion, though they do not feature in many psychiatric textbooks, are important in that respect, and they need not be tied to claims of exceptionalism. In Henry's case, religion seems to provide comfort but also a way of managing extreme feelings such as sinful guilt through praying, for example.

Henry also addresses the association between schizophrenia and violence, typical in media representations of mental illness, which became more prominent in the era of de-institutionalisation. His chapters in particular speak forcefully against the prolonged confinement to which he was subjected, even as his father exposes the problems of 'care in the community': the additional anxiety placed on families who could not care for their precarious members and how de-institutionalisation in the United Kingdom and the United States did not resolve the problem of stigma. Henry, who spent several years in secure wards, provides his own perspective: 'When people hear about a psychotic episode, they probably relate the word "psycho" to someone with violent tendencies. I would not describe myself as violent. I have really felt the strain of being in the hospital. Being locked up for so long really damages your spirits. You feel forgotten' (43). Henry criticises psychiatrists for having their 'own agenda' and not wanting 'to take risks' (222) and makes a pointed comment on the power dynamics between patients and professionals: '"I can hear what you are saying," said the psychiatrist, as, with the stroke of a pen, he renewed my section over my protests. I wondered if he realised what power he had in that pen. When it comes to being sectioned, what a professional psychiatrist says carries a lot of weight compared to that of somebody who has been diagnosed as a schizophrenic' (220).

Conclusion

In their provocative *BMJ* article, Patrick Bracken and Philip Thomas usher in a new era of 'postpsychiatry' that opens up 'the possibility of working with people in ways that render the experiences of psychosis meaningful rather than simply psychopathological' (Bracken and Thomas, 2001: 727). As they explain, postpsychiatry moves 'beyond the conflict between psychiatry and antipsychiatry' and rather than proposing 'new theories about madness' it 'argues that the voices of service users and survivors should now be centre stage' (Bracken and Thomas, 2001: 727). In their subsequent book, the authors outline a more detailed picture of postpsychiatry; its principal characteristics are 'dialogue', 'ethics before technology' and a holistic approach that pays attention to context (Bracken and Thomas, 2005: 1–21). Echoing Foucault, the authors write that 'if postpsychiatry means anything, it means an end to the "monologue of reason about madness"' (Bracken and Thomas, 2005: 2). Alongside other transformative illness narratives and cultural forms that explore such experiences, *Henry's Demons* demonstrates the important role memoirs can play in addressing the possibilities and challenges central to an era of postpsychiatry as well as in changing social attitudes toward disability.

On the question of recovery (poor outcome is still the variable most widely considered as a validating criterion for the diagnosis of schizophrenia), *Henry's Demons* adopts a realistic but not defeatist approach. There is no magical treatment to guarantee full recovery. Medication and therapy help but the urge to run away from hospitals stays with Henry. Henry's mother writes in her diary that often she feels like she is playing 'an unwinnable game of Snakes and Ladders' (139), which captures the difficulties experienced by caretakers and families. At the same time (and if we take away its pessimistic tone), the comparison suggests that even though schizophrenia may appear static because it is connected to a history of having been diagnosed with the condition, how one experiences it in reality can change over time. This is most evident in Henry's description of his 'polka-dot days', mentioned earlier in this chapter: 'I get the daemons or polka dots, which feel like a bad trip, about once a week, but they last less time than they used to, sometimes as little as two hours. When this happens, I just go to my bed and try and sleep them off' (221). This account shows that illness and health are not mutually exclusive, in other words that 'health within illness' is possible (Carel, 2008: 61).

Approaching our mental and emotional states as malleable and open to change forces us to give up whom Catherine Prendergast calls 'the stable schizophrenic, easy to incarcerate, or easy to celebrate as the occasion requires' (Prendergast, 2008: 61). A 'genuinely postmodern perspective', she writes, 'would not insist that schizophrenic rhetoric be fixed but rather would allow … to continue to engage in civic rhetoric, while being schizophrenic' (Prendergast, 2008: 61). There is no definitive closure for Henry and his story, as much as we may desire one. The book's final words are left to Henry. He says, 'It has been a very long road for me, but I think I'm entering the final straight. There is a tree I sit under in the garden in Lewisham which speaks to me and gives me hope' (222). This is approached by one reviewer as being 'as startling as the moment in a horror movie when the mutilated monster, long presumed dead, flicks open its green eyes' (Garner, 2011). I would rather approach it as an 'unexceptional' claim (to echo Prendergast) through which Henry continues to enjoy his rhetorical position as a narrator and his place in the public sphere, while being schizophrenic.

References

Bracken, P. and Thomas, P. (2005) *Postpsychiatry: Mental Health in a Postmodern World*, Oxford: Oxford University Press.

Bracken, P. and Thomas, P. (2001) Postpsychiatry: a new direction for mental health, *BMJ*, 322: 724–27.

Carel, H. (2008) *Illness: The Art of Living*, Durham: Acumen.

Cockburn, P. and Cockburn, H. (2011) *Henry's Demons, Living with Schizophrenia: A Father and Son's Story*, London: Simon and Schuster.

Couser, G.T. (1998) Making, taking, and faking lives: the ethics of collaborative life writing, *Style*, 32, 2, 334–50.

Couser, G.T. (2012) *Memoir: An Introduction*, Oxford: Oxford University Press.

Deleuze, G. and Guattari, F. (2009) *Anti-Oedipus: Capitalism and Schizophrenia*, London: Penguin.

Diedrich, L. (2007) *Treatments: Language, Politics, and the Culture of Illness*, Minneapolis: University of Minnesota Press.

Eakin, P. (1999) *How Our Lives Become Stories: Making Selves*, New York: Cornell University Press.

Egan, S. (1999) *Mirror Talk: Genres of Crisis in Contemporary Autobiography*, Chapel Hill: University of North Carolina Press.

Garner, D. (2011) Phantoms of the mind, no longer shocking but no less haunting, *The New York Times*, 1 February. Online. Available www.nytimes.com/2011/02/02/books/02book.html?_r=0 (accessed 2 July 2013).

Jameson, F. (1991) *Postmodernism, or, The Cultural Logic of Late Capitalism*, Durham: Duke University Press.

Laing, R.D. (1965) *The Divided Self: An Existential Study in Sanity and Madness*, Harmondsworth: Penguin.

Linklater, A. (2011) Henry's demons: living with schizophrenia, a father and son's story by Patrick and Henry Cockburn – review, *The Observer*, 20 February. Online. Available www.guardian.co.uk/books/2011/feb/20/henrys-demons-patrick-cockburn-review (accessed 2 July 2013).

Lovell, A. (1997) 'The city is my mother': narratives of schizophrenia and homelessness, *American Anthropologist*, 99, 2, 355–68.

Miller, N. (1996) *Bequest and Betrayal: Memoirs of a Parent's Death*, Bloomington: Indiana University Press.

Prendergast, C. (2008) The unexceptional schizophrenic: a post-postmodern introduction, *Journal of Literary and Cultural Disability Studies*, 2, 1, 56–62.

Radley, A. (2009) *Works of Illness: Narratives, Picturing and the Social Response to Serious Disease*, Ashby-de-la-Zouch: InkerMen Press.

Snyder, K., Gur, R., and Wasmer Andrews L. (2007) *Me, Myself, and Them: A Firsthand Account of One Young Person's Experience with Schizophrenia* (Adolescent Mental Health Initiative), Oxford: Oxford University Press.

Strauss, D. (2011) Two voices: Henry's demons, living with schizophrenia: A father and son's story, *The New York Times*, 11 February. Online. Available www.nytimes.com/2011/02/13/books/review/Strauss-t.html?pagewanted=all (accessed 2 July 2013).

Szasz, T. (1972) *The Myth of Mental Illness: Foundations of a Theory of Personal Conduct*, London: Paladin.

The Schizophrenia Commission (2012) *The Abandoned Illness: A Report*. Online. Available www.rethink.org/about-us/the-schizophrenia-commission (accessed 2 July 2013).

Thomas, P. (1997) *The Dialectics of Schizophrenia*, London: Free Association.

Woods, A. (2011) *The Sublime Object of Psychiatry: Schizophrenia in Clinical and Cultural Theory*, Oxford: Oxford University Press.

9   Impaired or empowered?

Mapping disability onto European literature

Pauline Eyre

In the world of disability scholarship, as a response to what David Bolt calls 'critical avoidance' (Bolt, 2012), a burning imperative has surfaced: to train scholars across the humanities to accord full value to the concept of disability, so that they come to consider its expression in cultural texts as the representation of something real, rather than assuming that it functions as merely a metaphorical mechanism to carry the thematic concerns of an author. This laudable drive to prepare a new generation of scholars is matched, however, by a persistent academic hunger for authors who are indeed capable of representing the complexities of disabled experience, whether through the raw experience of a life-writer or the intricately layered meanings laid down by a literary novelist.

A cultural model of disability no longer relies, of course, on pointing out the inadequacies of cultural artefacts in respect of people with impairments; rather, it seeks to celebrate exemplars of good practice across miscellaneous texts and media. Yet the predominantly Anglophone world of disability studies has thus far been impaired by a lack of engagement with the literature and culture of Europe where English is not the first language. This chapter, proceeding from a conviction that the net must be widened in the search for sophisticated representations of disability, investigates a novel written in German by a Czech writer – Libuše Moníková's *Pavane für eine verstorbene Infantin* (Pavane for a Dead Infanta; first published in 1983) – and argues that its exploration of a wheelchair user's life is of empowering importance to disability scholars, since it offers the kind of 'alternative way [...] of comprehending disabled bodies' for which Sharon Snyder and David Mitchell argue as a means of leaving behind objectifying research about disabled people (Snyder and Mitchell, 2006: 4).

Libuše Moníková (1945–1998) was born in Prague but spent most of her working life in Germany, developing a writing career alongside her university teaching jobs. *Pavane* is her second novel and although currently unavailable in translation, it urgently merits consideration by disability scholars on the basis of its challenge to the normal-disabled binary opposition. Significantly, Moníková always wrote in German rather than her native Czech, arguing that it gave her 'a necessary distance' (Kyncl, 2005) and it may be this sense of the insider-outsider figure at large in culture that provided her with the novel's starting point. *Pavane* is divided into two parts, the first of which describes the first-person narrator,

Francine's, sense of alienation, as a Czech emigrée who teaches literature at Göttingen University in Germany. Among her other problems, she has a painful hip. In Part Two, constituting a third of the novel's length, Francine adopts the use of a wheelchair, apparently as a reaction to her limp, and the reader accompanies her as she samples life as a disabled person, documenting both the positive and negative experiences this brings. Moníková also gives Francine an intellectual motive for taking to the wheelchair, namely an interest in disability as a literary theme (22) and in response to these twin motives she uses the wheelchair constantly over a period of months.

The first striking point of interest is, then, that the protagonist of this novel is a fraudulent wheelchair user, thus entering the novel into the debate about who has the right to represent people with disabilities. Is this not an affront to people with disabilities, in the same way that asking able-bodied actors to play disabled individuals is disempowering and reductive? My argument is that Moníková's supreme achievement in this novel is to get the nondisabled reader to identify with a disabled person precisely *because* the engagement with disability is temporary and non-confrontational. Neither pity nor sympathy is called for; there is no opportunity to leonise the heroic disabled person, no need to fall back on the notion of disabled characters as villainous. In short, this text does something radical: it represents the phenomenology of living as a disabled person without offering the reader a chance to render disability as Other.

Theoretical context

Hitherto, Moníková's novel has not been understood as a radical representation of disability. On the contrary, even Carol Poore's sustained and scholarly exploration of twentieth-century attitudes toward disability in German culture considers the text typical of a 'reductive discourse, which flattens out the real, lived experiences of disabled people' (Poore, 2007: 195–96). For the most part, *Pavane* has been read, like Moníková's other work, as an act of mourning for her Czech homeland (see, e.g., Braunbeck, 1997a) or seized on by feminists as a representation of female discomfiture within the constraints of patriarchy (Linklater, 2001; Gürtler, 2005). Indeed, feminism has provided the characteristic matrix for examination of Moníková's work. Until now, the wheelchair and the associated representation of disability within *Pavane* have been treated exclusively as metaphors that bolster the other themes of the text, most notably the protagonist's sense of alienation. The eminent German feminist and literary theorist Sigrid Weigel, for example, argues that Francine's painful hip is a psychosomatic expression of subjective conflict (Weigel, 1989: 122): she takes the wheelchair as no more than Francine's visible signal to the world of her psychological pain, a crutch par excellence.

My claim for *Pavane* as a dynamic representation of disability does not initially seem to be helped by examination of theoretical approaches to disability in Germany at the time of the book's publication. Whereas a vigorous intellectual offshoot had blossomed in the UK in parallel with the disability rights movement, the same was not true in West Germany. To a great extent, disability debate was hampered by a sense of national shame following World War Two, with the topic of disability provoking largely uncomfortable silence. People with disabilities simply dropped out of sight, still as strictly segregated from society as they had been under the National Socialist policies that ran alongside, and then superseded, the general euthanasia programme, abandoned in 1941 (Poore, 1982: 184). In consequence, disability discourse remained for a long time solely in the domain of the practical, the province of a select group of activists, rather than a matter for philosophical discussion among academic theorists. This situation hardly improved in the years leading up to Moníková's publication of *Pavane*: as late as 1980, a court in Frankfurt ruled in favour of a woman plaintiff who complained that her holiday had been ruined by the experience of having to share her hotel with a group of twenty-five disabled people. Astonishingly, she received an award for damages totalling half the cost of her holiday (Klee, 1980: 76). The resulting public outcry did nothing to overturn the court's ruling, but activist groups in West Germany now began to instigate targeted demonstrations aimed at raising the profile of people with disabilities.

The climate in which Moníková was writing, then, makes her choice of subject matter and protagonist all the more remarkable: at least part of the book's force lies in the fact that it predates the development of an academic disability agenda in German academia. What makes *Pavane* extraordinary is its systematic examination of the dynamics of existing as a disabled person. Against a societal background of routine incarceration of people with disabilities, Moníková sets in motion a disabled protagonist who is at large in the community, who documents experiences as she makes her way in the world, who monitors her own needs. Significantly, Moníková's heroine prefigures a model of self-determination (Selbstbestimmung), which surfaced in West Germany subsequent to *Pavane* (see, e.g., Steiner, 1999), but has much in common with Lennard Davis's notion of the dismodernist subject, whose impairments are central to subjectivity and yet fluctuate in value according to her or his current projects and her or his relationships of the moment (Davis, 2002).

Self-determination has much in common with the notion of independent living in the United Kingdom and United States, whereby the disabled individual becomes an employer with a degree of free will over the obtaining of personal assistance, but remains subject to the disciplinary practices of the neo-liberal society. In more recent times, this notion of self-determination has formed the basis of Anne Waldschmidt's 'flexible normalism' model of disability (Waldschmidt, 2006), an important contribution to German disability discourse that has steadily gained in authority, being showcased at disability conferences outside Germany (Chicago, May 2004; Lancaster UK, September 2006). According to this model, the disabled individual is required to oversee her or his own behaviour in the light of the behaviour of other individuals in the social group that situates her or him. Such self-monitoring practices result in a normal distribution curve based on an average that gives rise to a normalistic norm that adjusts dynamically. In Waldschmidt's model, there is no longer an opposition of normality and disability (Waldschmidt, 1998). Rather, the territory that accommodates both is shifting and variable: disability is reconfigured as a landscape that changes over time, being shaped by the disabled subject herself or himself, rather than constituting a category imposed by society.

This flexible normalist view of disability no doubt has its limitations, not least a tacit assumption that individuals with impairments subscribe to the same 'normal' values as those without disabilities. However, it promises a useful lens through which to view Moníková's novel where a disabled character is manipulated in such a way as to re-instate the experience of living in an impaired body as a fundamental, and normal, aspect of human experience. Moníková casts light on the relationship between individual impairment and the social category of disability; the possibility of existing as a modern, flexibly normal individual is interrogated; the relational variability of disability is exposed. In contrast to the normative reading strategies that have so far taken the disability represented in *Pavane* as merely a literary resource, thereby stripping the representation of its lived materiality, I am arguing that the novel should be read as a vibrant, phenomenological representation of disabled existence. My claim is based on an understanding of the entire text as a transliteration of Velázquez's celebrated painting, *Las Meninas* (which features a disabled woman in the foreground) and begins from the fact that Moníková insisted on a reproduction of the painting as the frontispiece for the first edition of *Pavane* (Mannsbrügge, 2002: 17). In subsequent paperback editions, a cropped version was used, to which pen and ink lines had been added, thus creating a personalised version of the painting to reflect the novel's thematisation of authenticity and authorship.

Las Meninas and *Pavane*: dabbling in disability

Perhaps it was Moníková's commitment to test the boundaries of fiction (Braunbeck, 1997b: 452) that led to her transliteration of Velázquez's painting, for she reproduced in her narrative all the themes that preoccupied her ground-breaking predecessor. Although this chapter does not offer the opportunity to examine its other themes, we should note that like *Las Meninas, Pavane* makes elaborate play with the business of looking at the world, drawing attention to the slipperiness of meaning; like Velázquez, Moníková toys with audience expectations, posing self and Other as interchangeable. On the left of the painting, an artist (said to resemble Velázquez himself) stands back from the canvas he is painting of King Philip IV and Queen Mariana, whom we see merely reflected in a small mirror in the background. The subjects of the portrait *we* see are the people watching the king and queen being painted: the eponymous maids-in-waiting, together with courtiers, a child with a dog, and a dwarf.

Velázquez often included in his paintings those disabled individuals who were customarily employed by the Spanish royal court as entertainers but also functioned as foils to the 'perfect' bodies of the royal household. Although appearing to comply with the Spanish convention of the period that social classes be represented in pyramidal form, ranging from royalty at the apex to children, animals, and people with disabilities at the base, Velázquez's prime motive in *Las*

Meninas is to undermine convention. True, the mirror in which the royal couple is reflected does indeed form the apex of a triangle whose base constitutes the 'baser' elements of sixteenth century society, including the disabled person. However, Velázquez's positioning of the disabled character in the foreground is a strategic manipulation of convention: crucially, the dwarf is nearest to the natural light from the window on the right hand side of the painting, a positioning that allows Velázquez to paint her naturalistically and with more candid detail than is seen elsewhere in the painting.

In committing to replicate Velázquez's sympathetic representation of an individual from a group often denied representation, Moníková pledges to undertake an intense investigation of the material nature of disability, systematically exposing the dynamics of disabled experience, such that the disabled person's point of view, her relationship with her body and her encounters with others, both disabled and nondisabled, are represented to an extent that is rarely encountered in fiction.

Moníková begins *Pavane* by representing Francine's experience of a painful hip as a simple impairment, a problem that is Francine's alone. In this section of the text, Francine notes from a position of 'normality' what it means to be disabled. Simultaneously pursuing her goal to thematise disability in literature (22) she notices blind people (45, 55), a woman with a walking stick (131), a disabled war veteran (74), wheelchair users (65, 110), and individuals with prosthetic limbs (44, 52), documenting not just their impairments but the compromises they make, their vulnerabilities and their manipulation of the social effects of their impairments. Importantly, Francine brings to her observations many of the stigmatising reservations that can structure nondisabled individuals' encounters with disability. Significantly, she finds that disability does not herald universally negative attitudes and experiences. While shopping, for instance, she notes that disabled people can expect undivided attention from smiling assistants, a state of affairs that is taken for granted by the woman using a wheelchair, who can expect the densest of crowds to part for her (64–65).

But it is Francine's encounter on a train with a young woman using a prosthetic leg that launches her interrogation proper of what it means to be disabled, and that is the ultimate spur to her experimental adoption of the role of 'disabled person' (52–53). Francine, entering the darkened sleeping coach of a train, stumbles over an artificial leg propped up in the corner. The conversation that ensues between the two women highlights many of the attitudes, misunderstandings, and uncertainties that characterise interactions between disabled and nondisabled individuals. For Francine, isolated and unhappy, the experience of being stuck in an awkward encounter with a disabled person is illuminating. Trying to control her own panic at confronting the woman's leg amputation, literally in the flesh, she notes the other woman's apparent ease and psychological advantage. By the time Francine rather sheepishly leaves the compartment she has registered a need to scrutinise more closely the comfortable hegemony of normality.

The beginning of Part Two of *Pavane* marks a transition. Fired by her goal of researching disability in literature and now recognising the symbolic power wielded by people who have been classed as disabled, particularly where the impairment is potently visible, Francine reconstructs herself as a disabled person and prepares to marshal her casual encounters with disabled people into a structured methodologically driven experiment. By launching Francine into the world with a highly visible accoutrement of disability, Moníková extends her interrogation beyond the world of private impairment into the public realm of disability. In recasting Francine as a disabled protagonist, Moníková re-assigns the malfunctioning body of her protagonist: it becomes a problem that is not hers alone but also impinges on the society around her. In particular, Moníková's project pivots on the trope of the wheelchair.

Toward a flexibly normal subject

The taboo-infringing mystery of a protagonist who fraudulently uses a wheelchair has taxed critical minds since the publication of *Pavane*. In my argument, the wheelchair is the linchpin of Moníková's novel, providing her with a means of linking the thematic concerns of the novel. First, it complies with the internal logic of the novel: delighted with her acquisition of the wheelchair, Francine explores its adjustable features and finds that her hip is free from pain when she sits in it (99). In other words, the adoption of the wheelchair temporarily removes Francine's impairment, so that she is able to 'disappear' into the other projects that occupy her over the course of the novel. This echoes Drew Leder's argument (1990) that the well body is normally absent when the subject is absorbed in projects: once Francine is equipped with a wheelchair, the 'absence' of the well body is restored; the wheelchair becomes incorporated into her subjectivity, no longer an object but 'an area of sensitivity' that extends her scope (Merleau-Ponty, 2002: 195).

Second, Francine's spurious adoption of the wheelchair provides Moníková with a focus for her transliteration of *Las Meninas*. By manipulating Francine as a would-be writer researching disability, Moníková draws attention to the synthesised experience of a disabled woman, probing the relationship between the materially impaired body and its cultural construction as a disabled body. In short, she interrogates the intersubjective nature of disabled being-in-the-world. I suggest that Francine is empowered by her use of the wheelchair. Yet there is a fundamental tension between the enabling properties of the wheelchair and its status as a highly visible signal to the world of the presence of gross impairment, a tension that Moníková exploits to the full. Functioning as the visual epitome of disability, the wheelchair serves to fix Francine's status as disabled, effacing other aspects of her subjectivity and providing the basis of her stigma at society's hands.

Typically, wheelchairs in literature have functioned as the kind of representational fetish described by Stuart Hall, whereby any feared category, such as disability, can be both indulged and disavowed (Hall, 1997). The reader of a novel featuring a wheelchair is encouraged to deny any connection between the trope of the wheelchair and the real malfunctioning body to which it is tethered. In other words, the wheelchair remains an empty metaphorical image to be treated solely as representational shorthand to support other themes in the text. Moníková knowingly exploits this fetishistic quality attached to the notion of a wheelchair, but perversely, it is the very inauthenticity of Francine's wheelchair pretence that allows Moníková to get behind the empty image and to facilitate a way for the 'aesthetically nervous' reader (Quayson, 2007) to identify, however temporarily, with the experience of a disabled person. In other words, she inveigles the reader into an encounter with the person who inhabits the wheelchair, inviting her or him to sample disabled experience from the inside, to experience alongside Francine the material reality of life as a disabled person.

Using the wheelchair, Francine learns to see the world differently: like any new adult wheelchair-user, she finds that life is practically very different; even her body is itself changed by wheelchair use (101). Crucially, Moníková exposes Western society as a normalised environment where the wheelchair user is repeatedly tested by exclusionary architectural practices. Without lifts, getting the wheelchair up to her apartment demands strength and persistence (126); without kerb-cuts, she must get out of the wheelchair or ask for help to mount the pavement; traffic is held up as she tries to extract her front wheel from a pothole (127). Francine is oppressed in other ways than merely by her surroundings. She is, for instance, subject to the illogicality of officious behaviour: she has a train ticket that is valid for a normal traveller but is told that, as a disabled person, she needs not a ticket but a free pass. Without it, the wheelchair counts as luggage and she must pay for it in addition to her ticket (106–107).

On the other hand, Moníková mischievously suggests that bureaucratic systems can work in disabled people's favour: Francine briefly considers applying for a professorial chair at the university, confident that her status as a wheelchair user would clinch the post for her. In other words, she comes to understand that disability need not simply mean compromise or a lowering of expectations; rather it can bring empowerment. Francine takes over the responsibility for identifying her own needs; wholeheartedly taking on the role of disabled person, she becomes an active consumer of disability products (109) rather than merely a passive recipient of benefits. It is entirely appropriate for her to consider buying stickers for her wheelchair (144) and to re-christen it her 'universal chair' (115) in an effort to remove the negative connotations she feels are associated with the traditional term.

Such acts of disabled agency reflect the notion of self-determination that has subsequently become the prime mode of thinking about disability in Germany. Francine becomes just the 'flexibly normal' individual whom Waldschmidt (1998) may have had in mind, writing some fifteen years after the publication of *Pavane*. Although responsibility for the impaired individual is in part shifted onto the social body, this model sees her accepted into the normal community with her membership contingent on both social conformity and on the wearing of a visible badge of her marginable status. The disabled individual is thus contracted to monitor her own behaviour according to rules that both empower her and render her responsible. Of course, a gap is now to be seen between the individual's experience of integration and the normal observer's tendency to re-marginalise her on the basis of the highly visible corrective equipment that she uses, here the wheelchair. For Francine, the wheelchair continues to influence people's treatment of her much more powerfully than does her facial expression (102).

By living as a disabled person, Francine becomes aware of the tensions in social attitudes toward disability. Indeed, Moníková demonstrates through Francine's experience that disability is not a category to be understood in opposition to normality: finding herself at the football stadium, Francine notes the row of wheelchairs behind the goal and, unused to the custom of seating wheelchair-using spectators together, she jumps to the conclusion that these are former footballers, invalided out of the game. Later, she realises that 'they can only be normal disabled people like me' (33). Moníková's deployment of the phrase *normal disabled* draws attention to the paramount objective of her work, namely the problematisation of boundaries. Francine is aligning herself, albeit pragmatically, with disabled people. The reader, unlike the people who encounter Francine within the narrative, takes her statement ironically, for her disability is fraudulent. The reader, in short, knows that she is not a 'normal disabled' person. Rather, she is 'normal'. Here, Moníková is exploiting the reader's fastidious separation of 'normal' and 'disabled' in order to expose the falsity of the distinction between them. Moníková's implication is that disability is a porous and flexible category. If Francine can function as both a normal and a disabled person, then by extension a disabled person's experience must be recognised as normal. Equally, occasions arise when normal people are disabled: Francine, for example, is more incapacitated by her experience of drunkenness in Part One of the novel (85–90) than she is by being a wheelchair user in Part Two.

Conclusion

Moníková's provocative and painstaking representation of disabled people's experience stages encounters that are not normally open to, indeed may be avoided by, the reading public. Thus, the personal interactions sedimented into a disabled person's experience are revealed in a systematic way that is not common in fiction. Moníková demonstrates that to be disabled is not to live as a fixed subject: disabled subjectivity is revealed as an open-ended set of potentialities where the meaning of disability varies moment by moment. Ultimately, disabled experience becomes detached from its customary mooring in the world of representational metaphor, so that it can be examined from a new perspective. If Merleau-Ponty argued that 'it is often a matter of surprise that the cripple or the invalid can put up with himself [sic], [t]he reason [being] that such people are not for themselves deformed or at death's door' (Merleau-Ponty, 2002: 504), then Moníková's achievement is to effect a situation where the disabled person is not deformed for the reader *either*, since by manipulating a protagonist who pretends disability, she forces the reader to inhabit both the disabled normality and the enabled abnormality of the impaired individual.

Moníková's project functions as a philosophical consideration of the cultural construction of disability. By undermining our impaired expectations of how disability can be represented, Moníková encourages the reader to temporarily take on the social role of an empowered disabled person. Her representation offers an invigorating examination of disabled experience, exposing the normalised disability experienced by so many disabled people who live as subjects and yet are gazed at as objects. *Pavane* provides a cogent example of how literary representation is not only capable of exploring the meanings attached to bodies, but is also a powerful tool to change those meanings.

Moníková's novel also drives home the point that the world of disability studies cannot afford to ignore German, or any other, literature. Indeed we need to insert all manner of texts into a cultural model of disability. By the same token, German scholars cannot afford *not* to engage with a cultural model of disability, even if that necessitates revising old readings of disability's presence in canonical texts. My findings allow hope, both for the empowering inclusion of material disabled experience in academic literary analysis and for recognition that fictional literature is an effective tool to change social attitudes toward disability.

References

Bolt, D. (2012) Social encounters, cultural representation and critical avoidance, in N. Watson, A. Roulstone, and C. Thomas (eds) *Routledge Handbook of Disability Studies*, London: Routledge.

Braunbeck, H.G. (1997a) The body of the nation: the texts of Libuše Moníková, *Monatshefte*, 89, 489–506.

Braunbeck, H.G. (1997b) Gespräche mit Libuše Moníková, 1992–1997, *Monatshefte*, 89, 452–67.

Davis, L.J. (2002) *Bending over Backwards: Disability, Dismodernism and Other Difficult Positions*, London: New York University Press.

Gürtler, C. (2005) Ihr Körper, neu zusammengestellt aus Begriffen, stand da. Körperbilder im Werk Libuše Moníkovás, in P. Broser and D. Pfeiferova (eds) *Hinter der Fassade: Libuše Moníková. Beiträge der internationalen germanistischen Tagung Ceske Budejovice – Budweis 2003*, Wien: Edition Praesens, 85–98.

Hall, S. (1997) The spectacle of the 'Other', in S. Hall (ed.) *Representation: Cultural Representations and Signifying Practices*, London: Sage Publications in association with the Open University.

Klee, E. (1980) *Behindert: Ein kritisches handbuch*. Frankfurt: S Fischer Verlag.

Kyncl, P. (2005) Libuše Moníková interviewed by Peter Kyncl: writing is a murderous occupation, in B. Haines and L. Marven (eds) *Libuše Moníková: In Memoriam*. Amsterdam: Rodopi.

Leder, D. (1990) *The Absent Body*, Chicago: Chicago University Press.

Linklater, B. (2001) 'Philomela's revenge': challenges to rape in recent writing in German. *German Life and Letters*, 54, 3, 253–71.

Mannsbrügge, A. (2002) *Autorkategorie und Gedächtnis: Lektüren zu Libuše Moníková*. Würzburg: Königshausen und Neumann.

Merleau-Ponty, M. (2002) *Phenomenology of Perception*, London: Routledge.

Moníková, L. (1988) *Pavane für eine verstorbene Infantin*, Berlin: Deutscher Taschenbuch Verlag GmbH.

Poore, C. (1982) Disability as disobedience? An essay on Germany in the aftermath of the United Nations year for people with disabilities, *New German Critique*, 27, 161–95.

Poore, C. (2007) *Disability in Twentieth-century German Culture*, Ann Arbor: University of Michigan Press.

Quayson, A. (2007) *Aesthetic Nervousness*, New York: Columbia University Press.

Snyder, S.L. and Mitchell, D.T. (2006) *Cultural Locations of Disability*, Chicago: University of Chicago Press.

Steiner, G. (1999) Selbsthilfe als politische Interessensvertretung, in E. Rohrmann and P. Günther (eds) *Soziale Selbsthilfe. Alternative, Ergänzung oder Methode sozialer Arbeit*, Heidelberg: Universitätsverlag, Ed. S.

Waldschmidt, A. (1998) Flexible normalisierung oder stabile Ausgrenzung: Veränderungen im Verhältnis Behinderung und normalität, *Soziale Probleme*, 9, 3–25.

Waldschmidt, A. (2006) Normalcy, bio-politics and disability: some remarks on the German disability discourse, *Disability Studies Quarterly*, 26, 2.

Weigel, S. (1989) *Die Stimme der Medusa: Schreibweisen in der Gegenwartsliteratur von Frauen*, Hamburg: Rowohlt.

10 The supremacy of sight

Aesthetics, representations, and attitudes

David Bolt

Representations of blindness have always been abundant in the cultural imagination. The trouble is that, though seemingly about blindness, these representations tend to focus on sight; indeed, they generally go so far as to endorse sight as the supreme sense, especially in relation to issues of aesthetics. This being so, cultural representations reveal much about social attitudes toward visual impairment. In this chapter I compare and contrast findings from two recent representational projects: the first focuses on literature and has been published in Canada as part of a *Mosaic* special issue on blindness (Bolt, 2013); the second focuses on advertising and has been published in the United Kingdom in a *British Journal of Visual Impairment* special on aesthetics (Bolt, 2014). In bringing together these projects, I consider the social attitudes toward visual impairment that are revealed in two very different forms of cultural text. The comparative aspect of the chapter is enhanced by the fact that the literary and advertising texts differ in their publication by more than a century.

The back-story

In the first of the two projects I coined the critical term *aesthetic blindness* to designate the highly problematic epistemological myth of blindness toward aesthetic qualities. Encapsulated in the term are a couple of erroneous yet commonplace preconceptions: that blindness is synonymous with ignorance and that aesthetic qualities are perceived by exclusively visual means. The representational and attitudinal problem that justifies this coinage is that blindness and aesthetics are often constructed so that the one is remote from the other, portrayed according to the supremacy of sight and thus incompatible with what I call visually impaired embodiment (i.e., a more inclusive approach to culture and society, whereby ocularcentric attitudes and assumptions are problematised if not dismissed).

The project's hypothesis was that aesthetic blindness was exemplified in literature from the 1890s, the era of the aesthete from which several blind characters sprang. In order to expand on this hunch I explored a number of works from the characteristically colourful, decadent decade with a focus on 1891, the year of Oscar Wilde's *The Picture of Dorian Gray*. I argued that, based on predominantly visual renderings of beauty and, by extension, knowledge, many of these representations of blindness focused on sight, meaning that the ontological status of the characters became diminished as they took on a ghostly form, an existence within yet without human society. That is to say, a blind Other was demarcated by an ocularcentric social aesthetic.

Maurice Maeterlinck's play *The Blind* (first published in 1891) was found notable for the way in which it immersed its audience and readers in aesthetic blindness; it made them concentrate on the value, if not imagine the necessity of sight in a social setting. Rendered in accordance with this ocularcentric social aesthetic, Maeterlinck's characters were burdensome, unproductive, devoid of empathy, and deficient in terms of both epistemology and ontology. These motifs were also found in works such as Rudyard Kipling's *The Light That Failed* and George Gissing's *New Grub Street* (both first published in 1891).

In the second of the two projects I turned to a recent advertising campaign. My interest was initially sparked when a producer of the BBC Radio 4 program *In Touch* invited me to speak on the subject in the summer of 2012. As a consequence I set out to develop a research instrument for the analysis of disability in advertising. Though relatively few, some critical studies of disability in twentieth-century advertising had already been conducted (Brolley and Anderson, 1986; Scott-Parker, 1989; Barnes, 1991; Ganahl and Arbuckle, 2001; Haller and Ralph, 2001; Panol and McBride, 2001; Thomas, 2001; Haller and Ralph, 2006), from which I extracted a problematic aesthetic. This sketch of bad practice was summed up in relation to issues of distortion; alterity; disclosure; segregation; and exclusion. The idea of the project was that the ableist aesthetic could be used as a model of representational regression against which advertisements would be measured.

In order to test the instrument I applied it to the twenty-first-century Dove Campaign for Real Beauty, inspired by the feminist critique that these advertisements are part of the very social aesthetic by which women become stereotyped and stigmatised (Dye, 2009; Froehlich, 2009; Johnston and Taylor, 2008; Scott and Cloud, 2008). In this work of feminist disability studies, I focused on three advertisements that featured women who have visual impairments: one for deodorant; another for the movement for self-esteem; and the other for hair colour radiance shampoo/conditioner. Aired between 2007 and 2012, all three advertisements were found to depart from the ableist aesthetic insofar as they contained slice of life representations and were used in a mainstream campaign. However, the supremacy of sight was not rejected entirely. These recent representations resonated with the aesthetic blindness that proliferated more than a century ago – a point on which I now expand.

The 1891 trilogy

In broad terms, in relation to visual impairment, the regressiveness of a representation (and its underpinning attitudes) can be assessed by its endorsement of sighted supremacy. This being so, Maeterlinck's *The Blind* constitutes a particularly regressive representation. Before the play commences, judging by its abundance of blind characters, not to mention its title, we might well infer that blindness is the main concern. However, set in the extraordinary darkness of an ancient forest, the play begins with the corpse of a *sighted* priest holding *centre* stage, on the right of whom there are six blind men seated on stones, tree-stumps, and dead leaves; on the left, separated from the men by more stones and a fallen tree, there are six blind women and a sighted baby. The gripping quality of this ocularcentric predicament, according to a late twentieth-century introduction to the play, rests in its very simplicity: 'The blind depend on the priest to see them to safety; the audience can see the priest is dead, though the blind cannot; so the blind are without succour, although they do not know it' (Slater, 1997: xv). There is little action, but dramatic tension results from the audience seeing what the characters cannot see, engaging in a 'teasing game of blindman's buff' with the characters 'stranded in sightlessness' (Gitter, 1999: 679). This privileging of sight is introduced in the exposition and expressed by the characters throughout the play.

Most strikingly, the supremacy of sight becomes manifest in a number of references to the aesthetic quality of the sun. Like the planets of our solar system, the conversation circles around the sun whose heat is nonetheless ignored in favour of its light. That is to say, their non-visual means of perception notwithstanding, the characters think of the sun in purely visual terms. The young blind girl reminisces about the fact that she has 'seen the sun' (22), both the oldest blind man and the oldest blind woman say that they have 'seen the sun' when they were 'very young' (17), whereas the third man born blind complains that he has 'never seen the sun' (17). Indeed, by modifying the verb *seen* with the adverb *never*, the third man born blind evokes a perplexingly profound sense of aesthetic exclusion, much as when the first man born blind dredges up the fact that they have 'never been able to see' (16) and the oldest blind man predicts, 'We'll never see each other' (31). The same exclusion is evoked when the young blind girl says that she has 'never seen' herself (24) and that she will 'never see' herself (31). Emphasised by repetition, the play's fixation on what has never been seen is indicative of the notion that aesthetic qualities are perceived by exclusively visual means.

Aesthetic blindness permeates the capacity for interpersonal relationships. The oldest blind man says:

> We've never seen each other. We ask each other questions, and we answer them; we live together, we're always together, but we don't know what we are! … It's all very well to touch each other with our two hands, eyes can see better than hands. (24)

Rather than conversation, shared experience, smell, sound, taste, touch, and so on, sight is the sole means by which he believes people get to know each other, a belief further illustrated when he adds, 'We've been together for years and years, and we've never had a sight of each other! It's as if we're always on our own' (25). In this ocularcentric social aesthetic, sight is required to validate the very existence of Self and Other and thus fundamental to any connection between the two, to the formation and function of human society.

The relational problem raises issues of compassion and community, for the blindness of Maeterlinck's characters 'strikes at the very heart of their being – it prevents them not only from seeing each other, but also from feeling for each other, from understanding each other, from loving each other' (Slater, 1997: xvi). Perpetuated by the claim that one must 'see to cry' (28), this assumption of emotional deficiency is taken to its extreme when the oldest blind man goes so far as to assert, 'You can't love someone without seeing them' (25), the dehumanising implication being that sightedness is a necessary condition of love. That is to say, Maeterlinck follows the age-old dramatic tradition of rendering blindness as symbolic castration.

Not only in drama, aesthetic blindness is also found in contemporaneously published works of realism such as Kipling's *The Light That Failed*. This novel tells the story of Dick Heldar, a painter who loses his sight as a result of a head injury sustained during his time as a war correspondent in Sudan. Prior to losing his sight he manages to complete his magnum opus, an oil painting called *The Melancholia*, which unbeknown to him is almost immediately defaced by its subject, Bessie Broke. This means that, as in Wilde's *The Picture of Dorian Gray*, the subject takes control over the art to which the artist thereby becomes oblivious. I make this assertion because Dick's idea of what is on the canvas in which he takes so much pride is manifestly erroneous. This example of aesthetic blindness is disrupted from time to time in the novel, such as when Dick is presented with the alternative of working with modelling wax, but sight remains paramount overall. The haptic aspect of aesthetics is dismissed by the artistic protagonist whose life thereby becomes meaningless; he is effectively a ghost of his former self.

Though ultimately pejorative, the construction of blindness in *The Light That Failed* is not as ocularcentric as Maeterlinck's *The Blind*. Like Maeterlinck's blind characters, Kipling's Dick Heldar comes to confuse day and night, 'dropping to sleep through sheer weariness at mid-day, and rising restless in the chill of the dawn' (167); however, when confused about the time, he would 'grope along the corridors of the chambers till he heard someone snore. Then he would know that the day had not yet come' (167). In other words, Dick's epistemology is informed by auditory as well as visual means, a multidimensional perspective that also has an aesthetic impact on his life. When longing for the sight of the moon, for example, he pauses to 'hear the desert talk' (206). The novel contains several such departures from aesthetic blindness, although we cannot help but notice the overall supremacy of sight, the idea that the light fails, soon to be followed by love, respect, art, beauty, and life itself. The depths of this pejorative representation are ploughed as the story ends with Dick returning to the battlefield and, as anticipated within and without the novel, getting killed.

A comparable but less prominent blind character can be found in Gissing's *New Grub Street*. Speaking very much of its time, this novel tells the story of a group of writers, editors, journalists, scholars, and other such literary folk. The group is said to be caught in a cultural crisis that hits Britain as universal education, popular journalism, and mass communication begin to have an impact on the literary community. Alfred Yule is the blind character in question, but his daughter Marian

Yule is the 'only completely admirable character' (Severn, 2010: 157). She works selflessly as a researcher and ghost-writer for her father until he loses his sight and thus his ability to be productive as an editor. She then takes financial responsibility for their family, works to the point of nervous breakdown, and as such reminds us of the centric role fulfilled by Maeterlinck's dead sighted character.

Like Maeterlinck's blind characters and Kipling's Dick Heldar, Gissing's Alfred Yule comes to endure an existence that is not only empty but also deemed burdensome. Readers are informed that, with blindness, there 'fell upon' Alfred the 'debility of premature old age' (414), that he 'might as well go home' and 'take his place meekly by the fireside', for he 'was beaten', soon to be a 'useless old man, a burden and annoyance to whosoever had pity on him' (335). This ocularcentric ontology is also portrayed by Kipling, for Dick is 'dead in the death of the blind, who, at the best, are only burdens upon their associates' (142). Because of the ocularcentric social aesthetic, both characters are judged parasitic. Their professional lives end because they have nothing left to give. Dick's life is 'nothing better than death' (167) and Alfred's is 'over' and 'wasted' (335). Indeed, when blind, Alfred becomes so insubstantial in relation to his former, sighted self that even his death is not narrated directly (Severn, 2010), but merely mentioned in passing at the dinner party with which *New Grub Street* closes: 'He died in the country somewhere, blind and fallen on evil days, poor old fellow' (420). This bleak end vividly illustrates the level of Otherness that can result from the ocularcentric social aesthetic.

The Dove trilogy

From what I have asserted thus far it follows that, in relation to visual impairment, the progressiveness of a representation (and its underpinning attitudes) can be assessed by its departure from sighted supremacy. This being so, on many levels the Dove trilogy is far more progressive than its 1891 predecessor. The literary texts are obviously far richer than their advertising successors but, judging by the manifestations of visually impaired embodiment, the underpinning social attitudes toward disability have become less ableist.

The deodorant advertisement, the first in the Dove trilogy, shows a woman who is alone but getting ready to go out with her friends. She asserts that she loves this chance to relax and pamper herself, that she finds the whole experience therapeutic. She explains that her deodorant and hair spray must be kept apart to avoid confusion between the two and thereby suggests that, for her, the purely visible labels are not accessible. This hint of visually impaired embodiment is sustained when we are told that the woman chooses her clothes by how they feel, that she has to be especially careful about using deodorant that leaves marks, and that she puts sellotape on the end of her eyeliner so as not to confuse it with lip liner. Her impairment finally becomes explicit when she asserts that she does most things by touch since losing her sight.

Despite the evidence of visually impaired embodiment, it is my contention that the initial concealment not only protects the normative aesthetic, but also adds punch to the revelation that the woman so preoccupied by looks does not perceive by visual means. The full power of this punch is captured in aesthetic blindness, the epistemological myth of blindness to aesthetic qualities, whereby visual impairment becomes synonymous with ignorance, and aesthetic qualities are perceived by purely visual means. After all, although the advertisement is for deodorant, the sense of smell is completely ignored. Indeed, aesthetic qualities perceived by other than visual means find expression, if not legitimation, via visual allusions and references. The woman says, 'I don't know why I use a mirror, I can't see myself', an expression of perplexity that is likely to spread to viewers, as the visual domain becomes appropriated by someone who perceives by other means. The use of the mirror resonates with aesthetic blindness, as though beauty must be assessed visually, a suggestion confirmed when the woman finally turns to the camera and asks, 'Do I look fit?' The importance of the visual assessment of her beauty thereby becomes explicit and viewers are offered a sense of narrative closure, a release from tensions around any suggested departure from the familiar ocularcentric aesthetic.

The movement for self-esteem advertisement, the second in the Dove trilogy, is similar insofar as it begins with a woman on her own, but she is not preoccupied with beauty or how she looks. Rather than getting ready for a night out, she is preparing for a game of cricket. The advertisement is also different because instead of concealing her visual impairment in order to reveal it as the narrative unfolds, this woman opens with an explicit reference to when she began to lose her sight. Indeed, where concealment is employed creatively in the first advertisement, in the second there may even be a charge of reductionism in the emphasis on visual impairment, a danger of 'reducing the complex person to a single attribute' (Garland-Thomson, 1997: 12). That said, although the woman reassures viewers that she has found her passion in the sport she plays twice a week, the vast majority of her direct speech refers or alludes to vision. So rendered, her situation takes on an ontologically insubstantial guise.

The advertisement is effectively fixated on vision and employs what is sometimes called an overcoming narrative (Mitchell and Snyder, 2000; Snyder and Mitchell, 2006). The woman employs ocularcentric language in order to overcome her visual impairment, to move on from when she began to lose her sight and – as in the setting of Maeterlinck's play – 'it all seemed so dark'. 'I found my passion', she asserts, 'I found the light'. At this point viewers see a sunlit scene that reveals the woman's passion to be cricket. The visual references continue as she says, 'I started to see things clearly' and 'I don't let my sight get in the way'. This contrary reference to 'sight' denotes visual impairment, which illustrates the point that 'if the actions of disabled individuals are cited as the source of overcoming, then it is only to the extent that they successfully distance themselves from the stigma of their own biologies' (Snyder and Mitchell, 2006: 208). The woman's self-esteem depends on her distancing herself from the stigma of her visual impairment. Paradoxically, then, this narrative about overcoming visual impairment works by rendering the woman's predicament in visual terms. But although the ocularcentric aesthetic ostensibly allows expression of achievement, it necessarily leaves those of us who have visual impairments Othered.

The advertisement for hair colour radiance shampoo/conditioner, the third in the Dove trilogy, also focuses on one woman, but represents a far more complex character. She is shown sitting on a sofa, in the shower, on the beach, in a car, in a boat, in a field, and so on. As in the first advertisement, the ableist aesthetic is not disrupted initially, for there are no signifiers of visual impairment until the woman finally says, 'Being blind I can't physically see the colour of my hair'. Thus, aesthetic blindness is implicit because, again, visual impairment is concealed for effect, specifically to bolster the revelation that a woman who both represents and has much to say about beauty does not perceive by visual means.

The main thing to note about the third advertisement is the evocation of wonder and Otherness that emanates from the concept of synaesthesia. In a radio discussion the creative director, Sarah Bamford, explains that the idea comes from a briefing with Dove and a colour psychologist about a test on someone who is blindfolded and yet can feel if colours are cool or warm (*In Touch*, 2012). Kate Crofts, the woman in the advertisement, asserts in the same programme that she is 'acutely aware of the synaesthesia phenomenon of enjoying and experiencing one sense through another' (*In Touch*, 2012). In the advertisement she tells viewers that colour is sounds, smells, and textures: yellow is sunshine on her face, lemon in her drink; blue is cool water, air, and sky. She also refers to the pertinence of different colours to different moods, a point problematically illustrated via an invocation of stereotypes, whereby blondes are 'bubbly and fun and girly' and red hair reveals passion. The supposed significance of colour becomes still more dramatic when viewers are told that even normal things become vivid: 'It's like the feeling of the sun on my skin or the wind in my hair'; 'I feel like laughing and dancing'; and 'I feel beautiful. It makes me happy and I want it to stay that way because I want to feel like that every day'. That is to say, she perceives by other than visual means but her very emotions are translated into visual terms. Indeed, the perception of colour becomes paramount, as though sight is the supreme sense by which the other senses are (and must be) led.

Conclusion

Though very different in their genres and separated by more than a century in their publication, the two representational trilogies unify in a number of ways. Most obviously, the 1891 trilogy brings together works from a key year in the decade of the aesthete, the Dove trilogy focuses on so-called real beauty, both employ blindness to make dramatic points about aesthetics, the supremacy of sight is a recurrent theme in all six individual texts, and people who have visual impairments effectively become Othered. In my work, in order to challenge and change the underpinning attitudes of these and other such representations, I posit a number of terms such as *aesthetic blindness, ocularcentric social aesthetic*, and *visually impaired embodiment*. My thesis is that, though fundamentally erroneous, aesthetic blindness results in an ocularcentric social aesthetic, a form of Othering that excludes those of us who do not perceive by visual means, but one that can be disrupted by expressions of visually impaired embodiment.

With this thesis in mind, we can also consider how the two representational trilogies differ, so as to speculate a little on how attitudes toward visual impairment have changed over the last century or so. Importantly, the fact that the women in the Dove trilogy all have visual impairments themselves indicates progressive attitudes insofar as the ocularcentric social aesthetic represented within the 1891 trilogy has not been sustained. That is to say, the Dove trilogy does not employ people who do not have visual impairments to play the parts of those who do. However, a note of caution on which I must end pertains to the fact that in film, radio, television, and theatre, the vast majority of actors who have played the blind characters in the various versions of works from the 1891 trilogy have not had visual impairments themselves. Indeed, when working on the present book I was approached to speak as an expert on representations of visual impairment at a new staging of Maeterlinck's play in the United States. I was flattered and initially agreed to contribute something, the premise of most of my work being that a key problem with representations of disability is the lack of informed critical engagement within literary and cultural studies. Thankfully, however, a colleague alerted me to my naivety about the staging in time for me to pull out. I had assumed the actors in this twenty-first-century project would themselves have visual impairments: alas, I was wrong.

References

Barnes, C. (1991) Discrimination: disabled people and the media, *Contact*, 70, 45–48.
Bolt, D. (2013) Aesthetic blindness: symbolism, realism, and reality, Mosaic, 46, 3, 93–108.
Bolt, D. (2014) An advertising aesthetic: real beauty and visual impairment, *British Journal of Visual Impairment*, 32, 1.
Brolley, D. and Anderson, S. (1986) Advertising and attitudes, in M. Nagler (ed.), *Perspectives on Disability*, Palo Alto: Health Markets Research.
Dye, L. (2009) A critique of Dove's Campaign for Real Beauty. *Canadian Journal of Media Studies*, 5, 1, 114–28.
Froehlich, K. (2009) Dove: changing the face of beauty? *Fresh Ink: Essays From Boston College's First-Year Writing Seminar*, 12, 2.
Ganahl, D.J. and Arbuckle, M. (2001) The exclusion of persons with physical disabilities from prime time television advertising: a two-years quantitative analysis, *Disability Studies Quarterly*, 21.
Garland-Thomson, R. (1997) *Extraordinary Bodies: Figuring Physical Disability in American Culture and Literature*, New York: Columbia University Press.
Gissing, G. (1996) *New Grub Street*, Hertfordshire: Wordsworth.
Gitter, E.G. (1999) The blind daughter in Charles Dickens's 'Cricket on the Hearth', *Studies in English Literature, 1500–1900*, 39, 4, 675–89.
Haller, B. and Ralph, S. (2001) Profitability, diversity and disability: images in advertising in the United States of America and Great Britain, *Disability Studies Quarterly*, 21.
Haller, B. and Ralph, S. (2006) Are disability images in advertising becoming bold and daring? An analysis of prominent themes in US and UK campaigns, *Disability Studies Quarterly*, 26, 3.
In Touch. (2012) BBC Radio 4. 24 July 2012.

Johnston, J. and Taylor, J. (2008) Feminist consumerism and fat activists: a comparative study of grassroots activism and the Dove Real Beauty Campaign, *Journal of Women in Culture and Society*, 33, 4, 941–66.

Kipling, R. (1988) *The Light That Failed*, London: Penguin.

Maeterlinck, M. (1997) *Three Pre-Surrealist Plays*, Oxford: Oxford University Press.

Mitchell, D.T. and Snyder, S.L. (2000) *Narrative Prosthesis: Disability and the Dependencies of Discourse*, Ann Arbor: University of Michigan Press.

Panol, Z.S. and McBride, M. (2001) Disability images in print advertising: exploring attitudinal impact issues, *Disability Studies Quarterly*, 21.

Scott, J. and Cloud, N. (2008) Reaffirming the ideal: a focus group analysis of the Campaign for Real Beauty, *Advertising and Society Review*, 9, 4.

Scott-Parker, S. (1989) *They Aren't in the Brief: Advertising People with Disabilities*, London: King's Fund Centre.

Severn, S.E. (2010) Quasi-professional culture, conservative ideology, and the narrative structure of George Gissing's *New Grub Street*, *Journal of Narrative Theory*, 40, 2, 156–88.

Slater, M. (1997) Introduction, in M. Maeterlinck *Three Pre-Surrealist Plays*, Oxford: Oxford University Press.

Snyder, S.L. and Mitchell, D.T. (2006) *Cultural Locations of Disability*, Chicago: University of Chicago Press.

Thomas, L. (2001) Disability is not so beautiful: a semiotic analysis of advertising for rehabilitation goods, *Disability Studies Quarterly*, 21.

Part III

Disability, attitudes, and education

11 Ethnic cleansing?

Disability and the colonisation of the intranet

Alan Hodkinson

This chapter formalises my thoughts in relation to the electronic media emplaced in schools' intranet sites. These sites are re-drawn as ontological envelopes. Such envelopes enfold, constrict, and constrain individualisation. They form and malform societal attitudes through 'impoverished representations' (Latour, 2010: 44), sealing the 'smoothed' out images within totalising structures of modern power and ableist agendas (Agamben, 1998). I re-think schools' intranet sites, recasting them as 'covert forms of manipulation' where pronominal games and illocutionary mirrors reflect an imposed lexis and unresolved dialectic between constituting and constituted power (Pinto, 2004). An examination of these intranet sites reveals the imposed binary dialectics and unearths 'the conditions of exclusion experienced by people with impairments' (Goodley, 2007: 145). In education, such dialectical oscillations and 'rules of civility' striate individual bodies, societal attitudes, freedom, and social justice as the information communicated through intranet sites imposes semiotic coordinates, which 'maintain a delicate balance between modest imprecision and mannerist stereotype' (Agamben, 1998: 58). In this space of mistranslation, representations of the 'impaired organism' are bound within hierarchical organisation – signified through structured systems of organisational control, language, and images – that subjectifies the disabled individual as Other.

I first engaged in this research after a teacher informed me that the school's intranet site provided a safe space for children to learn. Subsequent analysis of such safe spaces revealed artefacts of disability that were limited and contextualised by medical deficit. These artefacts formed a social construction of disability (based on inexact scholarship, omission, and imbalanced information), where negative conceptualisations, enabled perhaps by stereotypical attitudes, colonised the electronic landscape.

As I set out to explore this territorialisation my intellectual endeavour became the examination of the cultural image of individuals and communities in the intranet space. The endeavour led me to historical archaeology as a technique to provide a theoretic grounding for analysing how identity is formed and malformed within such spaces. Historical archaeology is an innovative, improvisational, and context dependant method that seeks to examine the 'dominant group's sense of "self"' (Chapman et al., 1989: 19). This method formulates alternate means of pursuing the archaeology of marginalised groups by seeking to 'ironicize master narratives' (Funari et al., 1999: 17). Historical archaeology's exploitation of the mosaic of the traditional disciplines of archaeology and ethnography (Meskell, 2007) provides explanatory mechanisms of property and processes that enable simple correlates between materials and so-called static phenomenon to be provided (Roux, 2007). This methodology does not assume that living people are frozen relics of the past, but rather that strands of connection exist between past and living communities (Meskell, 2007).

The electronic media placed on schools' intranet sites became my static artefacts. They were the link between the intranet present and a pre-intranet past. These artefacts enabled a temporal, spatial, and historical analysis of the societal conceptualisation and attitudes toward disability to be countenanced. This chapter seeks to better illuminate the images, conceptualisations, and attitudes toward disability left by the colonisers of this intranet space. I, like Petra Kuppers, seek to 'subvert the structural position of "disability" as a marker' (Kuppers, 2003: 4). I likewise want to reveal how societal attitudes and representations of illness and disability 'contain the Other, [they] isolate it, present it outside "normal" society and bodies' (Kuppers, 2003: 4).

The plantation settlement and the colonising of space

Landscapes are topologies of relationships that, ethnologists argue, have utility and relevance to the ways in which the past and present are embedded in culturally informed practices (Whitehead et al., 2010). The prima facie concern of the ethnologist is to decipher 'the manner in which a place is organised' by paying close attention to the layout of villages and their arrangements of house and to observe these constructs as a transcription of space (Auge, 1995: 42). Analysis of colonial cartographies (Whitehead et al., 2010), such as the one I forward here, must interpret the non-tactile dimensions of social practices such as the arrangement of buildings (Pels, 1997). The argument in this chapter is that within these schools' intranet sites the administrative control of the plantation settlement re-materialised. This organisational control, I suggest, became the strong point of occupation that (as in European colonisation) provided the model for the enslavement of this society's conceptualisation and attitudes toward disability (Pels, 1997). My analysis, then, recast me as the ethnologist who, following the missionaries and first waves of settlers, aimed to decipher the geography and people of this new space and digital age (Auge, 1995).

My exploration of schools' intranet sites highlighted a space of ordered regularity and conventional geometry (see Figure 11.1). As I gazed at the computer screen, small yellow folders shone forth. These were organised in serried ranks bounded by neat rows and columns of ordered space. Each intranet site was formulated within a hierarchical structure. Invariably, the first folder emplaced was labelled to represent a core National Curriculum subject – usually literacy or numeracy. This was always closely followed by science. Subsequent organisation was less ordered but normally involved the foundation subjects of history,

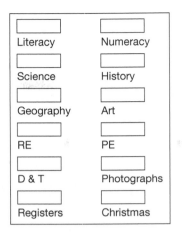

Figure 11.1 Layout of the plantation settlements

geography, religious education, and so on. After this the folders became more random, including such things as Christmas, school forms, school pictures or registers. The more I observed these yellow folders, these portmanteaus of organisation, the more they resembled the order of my old school filing cabinet. This battered grey cubicle of space occupied the corner of my classroom, silently maintaining control of paper copies of curriculum material and the general detritus of school life. The system of ordering on the intranet sites was the same as in the filing cabinet. This was a map of a landscape engraved on teachers' souls (Bachelard, 1994). As I further observed these folders they appeared to me as the roofs of houses, surrounded by neat and ordered streets. To employ the words of Bachelard, we might say a 'past history had come to dwell in these new houses' (Bachelard, 1994: 10).

My field notes of this landscape demarcated a managed garden, rather than a pasture wilderness, where the synergy of habitat and people produced a physical and intellectual context for analysis (Whitehead et al., 2010). The organisational structure of these plantation settlements dominated the intranet space. This space had witnessed a 'concrete ritual of emplacement' that appeared to reaffirm and reinstate old world orders (Auge 1995: 5). In these plantation settlements, the house had become the corner of this world (Bachelard, 1994). This intranet village, though, was not in Bourdieu's terms a paradigmatically silent habitus (Shields, 1997). Rather, in this manifestation of society, highly stratified settlement patterns were observable (Whitehead et al., 2010). Literacy and numeracy acted ideologically as the planter's mansion. These subjects dominated the organisational high ground, impacting on social and educational processes, as in colonial plantation settlements. The foundation subjects and other school materials were relegated and set aside as plantation shacks, controlled from above and subservient to the core subjects.

Plantations have been defined as the literal planting of people into new ground in the establishment of settlements (Radune, 2005) and discrete spatially bounded sites whose patterns of settlements reflected a system of centralised control (Orser, 1990). My attention, though, focused on plantations as 'symbolic representations' that expressed power and control through 'settlement patterning' (Joseph, 1993: 59). Here, it seemed that, through 'carefully constructed landscapes', the planter 'geographically located' (Joseph, 1993: 59) and 'actively constructed plantation spaces' (Delle, 1999: 136) as an altar of control, enabling the development of Omnipotent relations on the plantation and beyond (Orser, 1990). This plantation ideology enabled a reference point of how teachers ordered and controlled the intranet space. Within these bounded spaces and processes of colonisation, as those residing in the plantation huts, the image of the inhabitant was also heavily controlled.

Pausing here to reconsider historical archaeology, I find it interesting to note that its central focus is the analysis of complex power relationships expressed in terms of concepts such as domination/resistance, inequality, and colonisers/colonised (Funari et al., 1999). However, we should not forget that the main battleground of colonialism was the control of land and the implanting of settlements (Said, 1993). Colonisation was not just about 'soldiers and cannons', but also 'forms, about images and imaginings' (Said, 1993: xxi). In these terrains of dialectic and praxis, the raison d'être of colonialism resided in its 'power to narrate, or to block other narratives' (Said, 1993: xii) and to form and reform attitudes toward indigenous people. The 'power to represent the nation is already the power to dominate it' (Larsen, 2000: 40). Colonialism, then, is always centred on managing heterogeneity and dealing with difference by 'imposition, restriction, regulation and repression' (Quayson, 2000: 112).

In some views, complexity is inevitable in the cultural and social entailments of ethnographic phenomena such as colonialism (Strathern, 1991), but only through simplification can complexity truly be revealed (see Quayson, 2000). Accordingly, I detail what at one level is a simple analysis of the artefact of disability unearthed within intranet spaces. However, this analysis is also complex as it captures the processes of colonisation in action. Such processes provide the critical foregrounding to a phenomenological shrinkage (Larsen, 2000) of the 'ontological inscription of otherness' into this electronic geography (Quayson, 2000: 100). I seek to move away from analysis of the electronic environ as a 'domain of things' to a discussion that embraces the images and 'ways of thinking' bound up in the processes of colonisation (Quayson, 2000: 100). My argument is relatively simple, that the artefact of disability may be read as a social text, the semioses of which stands in place of an institutional consciousness, substituting extant discourses of practices (Larsen, 2000) for a sanitised telos. The complexity of cultural and social entailments formed here, then, relies on a telos that obviates the Disability Rights Agenda through the imposition of ideological misrepresentations (Larsen, 2000). These artefacts, bounded within the power discourse of the plantation settlements, revealed the enslavement of the history of disability by rendering it as subaltern of the white, able-bodied male. Positive attitudes and images of disability within these internet spaces became a banished ghost, destined to roam at the margins of society (Larsen, 2000).

'Enslavement' of the image of disability

The images within the colonised space are noteworthy in several respects. The major finding of this research was the virtual absence of an image of disabled people. Of the 4,485 illustrations, 930 photographs, and 59 video clips analysed, only 34 images represented disability, of which the commonly portrayed picture was physical disability. Indeed, no textual reference to, or pictures of, intellectual disabilities were observed: 26.5 per cent of these images portrayed wheelchair users, of which only 8.8 per cent were independent users; 7.7 per cent showed people with a limb amputation; and 11.7 per cent located disability within the image of a pirate. Also of interest was the fact that only 8.8 per cent of the images located disability in the image of a child (less than 0.05 per cent of the total images analysed). It was particularly concerning that only two images represented positive images of disability. A major finding from the study was that in the wealth of school images analysed – such as playgrounds, classrooms, swimming lessons and school sports days – no picture of disability was observable. The finding highlighted that the most prevalent image to which the school children we introduced was that of the white, non-disabled adult male.

In the linguistic analysis only two pieces of texts referring to disability we uncovered. First, in an electronic storybook, disability as metaphor was construc through the image of a pirate (a not uncommon image in the dataset). The chara concerned was employed to represent the 'baddy' in the narrative. The pirat this pictorial form was a diminutive figure; rather overweight and with ru cheeks, he did not look in the best of health. Indeed, some would say he looke though a heart attack was imminent. He had a lower limb amputation, a prostl limb made out of wood, a visual impairment necessitating an eye patch, a 'scruffy black beard' (Lawson, 2006). The description stated:

> Of course like most pirates [he] had a wooden peg for a leg so every no
> then he would wobble and hobble as he walked …
>   All in all [he] didn't seem like a very fearsome pirate at all.
>
>   (Lawson

Here, the image of disability was constructed through a person suppose 'sinister and evil'; however, this pirate could not even get that characte right. Instead, he was located within the text more as a pitiable and pathetic an object of ridicule (Barnes and Mercer, 2003).

It is important to remember here that, throughout the history of western physical disabilities such as a so-called hunched back, a hook, a wooder an eye-patch have been employed as metaphor for evil and depravity (C Bejoian, 2007). In contrast, 'goodness' is articulated by angel-like fig long flowing locks and smiling faces. Such dichotomous images tell deal about a society, its attitudes and its values (Connor and Bejoian, 20 images, then, may be observed as a form of disablism leading to the abno of the cultural image and negative attitudes toward disabled people.

In the second example, an electronic science textbook employed an image of an occupational health therapist showing a wheelchair to a child. A caption under the image read, 'Occupational therapists help children with disabilities to be as independent as possible. They also help if you go back to school after a long illness or severe injury'. Disability here was located as medical deficit through the use of words such as *injury* and *illness*. We should also pause to note both that occupational therapists *help* children with disabilities and the use of the conjunction *if* in relation to them going back to school'. This text elevated quasi medical professionals into positions of power and control over people with impairments; it did not promote a positive image nor attitude toward disability, but rather served to highlight the power dynamics involved in 'therapeutic care'; and it seemingly made plain who controlled the decision of whether a child is allowed back into school.

The unearthing of this artefact of disability does not in Matthew Arnold's terms provide a 'reservoir of the best that has been known and thought' (cited in Said, 1993: xiii). Rather it produces 'registers of assumptions' and 'efficacious signs of identification' where the 'ontological inscription of otherness' is (mal)formed within a hierarchical and variegated demography (Quayson, 2000: 100). Analysis of this aestheticised and commodified artefact of disability, bounded within plantation ideology, reveals the process of colonialism at work. Missionary teachers controlled the 'system representing as well as speaking for everything within its dominion' (Said, 1993: 13). Ontologically speaking, the process of colonisation emplaced here provides a social text of 'unchanging intellectual monuments' of disability that legitimised a grand narrative of ableism (Said, 1993: 12). This discourse of modernity bears witness to 'a mental attitude of the colonist', the 'inability to conceive of any alternative', thus revealing the formulation and control of the demographic (Fieldhouse cited in Said, 1993: 13). Within this terrain, the teachers may be observed as a 'repressive force' that excluded the heterogeneity of past ages, recasting the ancestors, the strong and positive image of disability, within an institutional homogeneity of normalisation and ableism (Quayson, 2000).

Discussion

The data evidenced here provide a narrative to the creation of a space of possibilities and how this *chora* became striated into Euclidean space by missionary teachers who colonised this undiscovered brave new world – a world that offered the prospect that disability may have become located within a new cultural framework. After all, 'what can be more sublime than the creation of a liberated territory of positive order of being which escapes the grasp of the existing order' (Žižek, 2009: 116)? Problematically, while the colonial power ensured this world was safe from pornography and paedophiles, other aspects of colonisation were not subject to similar 'control orders'. The intranet here became an anti-democratic space controlled by a colonising power that employed an axis mundi of 'selective tradition' (Williams, 1961) to striate, subjugate, and delineate electronic space with old world orders. Teachers, recast as missionaries, delivered a 'civilising and repressive force' reminiscent of Victorian cultural imperialism as they took up special positions 'at the juncture of colonial technologies of domination and self-control' (Pels, 1997: 168). They became the masterful and pioneering power that codified, channelled, and regulated intranet space (Deleuze and Guattari, 1972). In creating *their* modernity of space they built plantations of knowledge and identities whose architecture was domination and whose building materials were technologies of self (Van der Veer, 1995). As in the late 1800s, missionary zeal here produced a 'civilised' (in their eyes at least) image of a disabled indigene fit to be observed by the wave of subsequent settlers: the children who entered and explored this world in the name of education. This expropriation of space left permanent legacies of an internal colonialism, of hegemony based on the sanitisation of the image of the Other (Pels, 1997).

The uncovering of this artefact of disability felt uncomfortable. It raised the spectre that a process of ethnic (or perhaps cultural) cleansing had been quietly and privately accomplished. It appeared that a genome, a media project, had swept through this space, clearing a terra nullius – a 'land that belonged to nobody' (Meekosha, 2011: 672). Expulsion of some settlers (the new indigenes) as illegal immigrants produced a private environ (Auge, 1995) whose residual artefact was a social hieroglyph of disability formed within a cultural cloak of bigotry and psycho-medical pejorative traditions. As in Vietnam, after the expulsion of the American army, the ancestor spirits were re-categorised by the conquering force and so a strong ancestry of disability rights was relegated to the status of the *ang bac* (ghost) and thrown out from the new plantation settlements (Kwon, n.d.). Societal control exercised in line with that of the Mexican Instituto Nacional de Antropología e Historia sanitised the artefact of the indigene, moulding it to inculcate settlers into a hegemony of an ableist society. This artefact of disability (its residual hieroglyph) became the hidden-away refugee of equality. This Foucauldian leper was non-threatening, subjugated, and controlled, and placement at the borders of the new striated space was observed as acceptable. The intranet space, then, had been subject to a territorialisation (Deleuze and Guattari, 1987). I realised that disability had become Pavlov-West's (2009) 'Irish theme pub'. Within this territory, then, a chain of clones, a recreated, reconceptualised essence and attitude toward disability, of being and belonging, was mapped out within the fallacious architecture of the rustic model village. In this formalised culture a motif of reduction operated that made present 'an easily assimilable version of a complex reality' (David, 2001: 141), while absenting the concrete reality of impairment based upon an ontological assumption (see Chiesa, 2009).

The narrative of this new world is both dark and oppressive. However, I now suggest how control of this 'disabling' narrative might be reclaimed *by* and *for* all who wander this digital topography. I sketch out a new cartography where the colonial mansions and plantation settlements are dismantled. In line with the *utopia of hope* (Bloch, 1995), closed systems of oppression would be opened up and re-framed. This future landscape – this not-yet-consciousness (Bloch, 1995) – would observe the creation of a homeland of social justice where equality would stand as an achievable state and as an alternate possibility to the created 'rational' electronic society that now exits. The reforms I detail articulate my own 'wishful images' (Bloch, 1995).

Education in this landscape would be reframed within the principles of human rights, democracy, equity, and social justice. The ultimate aim of digital media and internet technology would be to develop schools' intranet sites where all children could participate and be treated equally, and where the imperative would be developing positive social attitudes toward disability (Sandhill, 2005). In converting this aim into reality the imperative is that all material located in this electronic space must address discrimination, equality, and 'the status of vulnerable groups in society' (Sandhill, 2005: 1). Paradoxically, I contend that more control/censorship of this 'great space of internet democracy' might bring forth education that is more culturally sensitive. In this form, education would become a moral concept necessitating the expression of the values of self-fulfilment, self-determination, and equality. However, a pre-requisite to the promotion of cultural democracy is that the individual has the right to participate and to be included at a social, intellectual, and cultural level (Bernstein, 1996). For this new space to become effective the control of the intranet by teachers has to be challenged. Schools have to recognise that relations of dominance exist in society and that obstacles to effective education have become embedded in simple everyday habits of this new electronic world (Slee, 2001). My belief is that if this world is to move beyond the 'phenomena of structure' (Clough, 2005: 74), building upon human rights and the democratic imperative, it must give preference to strategies of empowerment and the development of positive attitudes toward disability. It is in this democratic imperative that the mediating role of the electronic media within pedagogical space becomes important. This space is within our grasp, but we need to reach out and take it one keystroke at a time.

Conclusion

Within the virtual space, the missionary teachers and colonial government had a unique opportunity to move beyond 'post-modern local narratives' and disturb their functions by producing a truth that intervened in the Real, perhaps causing 'it to change from within' (Žižek, 2009: 33). Here was a new space of politic and possibilities, a chance to create a democratic, emancipatory, and perhaps even subversive world. However, the missionaries' colonisation subjugated and striated this intranet space, collapsing it for a 'multitude of oscillations into a reality based on the reduction of open space' (Chiesa, 2009: 210). Deciphering of the organisation and representation of the 'disabled indigene', through the theoretical framework of historical archaeology and colonialism, unearthed a cartography inscribed by a scalpel of the old world geometry and ableist attitudes (Deleuze and Guattari, 1987). Colonisation, acting as the 'overcoding machine' (Deleuze and Guattari, 1987), produced a 'geometrico' of homogeneous space that determined the substance, form, and relations of the electronic environ. Disability, synthesised into this reality, became the Deleuzian virtual shadow of its former ideological self. This locality, then, did not separate figures from affectations. Rather it (re-in)forced morphological formulations as the primacy of the theorem element where people with impairments became segments of their segmentations (Deleuze and Guattari, 1987). This new world, predicated on extant Lacanian Master-Signifier relationships, was founded upon 'ground rules' that were 'grounded only in themselves' (Žižek, 2009: 22). Thus, images captured within plantation ideology, and overcoded by old world geometry, empowered phenomenological reduction and the 'homogenising logic of the institution' to '(re)produce a homogeneity of demographic' (Golberg, 2000: 73), hollowing out this space as a site of emancipatory possibilities (Larsen, 2000; Žižek, 2009). This framing of disability, its residual artefact, therefore, hid from view 'differences and distinctions' that 'flowed through the heart of the colonizing darkness' (Golberg, 2000: 73). 'Homogenising the heterogeneous', it fixed the 'flow and flux' with a praxis that rendered passive the strong and positive image of the ancestors (Golberg, 2000: 84). This colonised world rejected subjective experience and object materialism (Žižek, 2008), and constructed disability as a 'staged cultural reality of mental states or perhaps behavioural dispositions to all' (Benthall, 2008: 1).

The silence of the ancestors is deeply troubling, as initial ignoring (or perhaps lack of veneration) ultimately renders these indigenes as invisible (Golberg, 2000). For Said, the wonder of such 'representational exceptionalism' (Golberg, 2000) is that schooling becomes provisional in its outlook and action, 'unchecked, uncritically accepted, recurring, replicated in the education of generation after generation' (Said, 1993: 20). I must ask if the settlers of this new world – the children exploring these environs – are repeatedly presented with such ideological formations, what effect will it have on their attitudes toward disability?

References

Auge, M. (1995) *Non-places: Introduction to an Anthropology of Supermodernity*, London: Verso.

Agamben, G. (1998) *HOMO SACER, Sovereign Power and Bare Life*, California: Stanford University Press.

Bachelard, G. (1994) *The Poetics of Space*, Boston: Becon Press.

Barnes, C. and Mercer, G. (2003) *Disability*, Cambridge: Polity.

Benthall, S. (2008) *Popper's Third World*. Online. Available http://interrationale.wordpress. com/popper (accessed 6 September 2013).

Bernstein, B. (1996) *Pedagogy, Symbolic Control And Identity: Theory, Research, Critique*, London: Taylor Francis.

Bloch, E. (1995) *The Principle of Hope*, volume 2, Cambridge: MIT Press.

Chapman, M., McDonald, M. and Tonkin, E. (1989) Introduction, in E. Tonkin, M. McDonald, and M. Chapman (eds) *History and Ethnicity*, London: Routledge.

Chiesa, L. (2009) The world of desire: Lacan between evolutionary biology and psychoanalytic theory, *The Yearbook of Comparative Literature*, 55, 200–25.

Clough, P. (2005) Exclusive tendencies: concepts, consciousness and curriculum in the project of inclusion, in M. Nind, R. Rix, K. Sheey, and K. Simmons (eds) *Curriculum and Pedagogy in Inclusive Education: Values into Practice*, Buckingham: OUP.

Connor, D. and Bejoian, L. (2007) Crippling school curricula: 20 ways to teach disability, The *Review of Disability Studies: An International Journal*, 3, 3, 3–13.

David, R. (2001) Representing the Inuit in contemporary British and Canadian juvenile non-fiction, *Children's Literature in Education*, 32, 139–53.

Deleuze, G. and Guattari, F. (1972) *Anti-Oedipus: Capitalism and Schizophrenia*, New York: Viking.

Deleuze, G. and Guattari, F. (1987) *A Thousand Plateaus*, London: Continuum.

Delle, J. (1999) The landscapes of class negotiation on coffee plantations in the Blue Mountains of Jamaica: 1790–1850, *Historical Archaeology*, 33, 1, 136–58.

Funari, P.A., Jones, S., and Hall, M. (1999) Introduction: archaeology in history, in P. Funari, S. Jones, and M. Hall (eds) *Historical Archaeology – Back from the Edge*, London: Routledge.

Golberg, D.T. (2000) Heterogenity and hybridity: colonial legacy, postcolonial heresy, in H. Schwarz and S. Ray (eds) *A Companion to Postcolonial Studies*, London: Blackwell.

Goodley, D. (2007) Becoming rhizomatic parents: Deleuze, Guattari and disabled babies, *Disability and Society*, 22, 2, 145–60.

Joseph, J.W. (1993) White columns and black hands: class and classification in the plantation ideology of the Georgia and South Carolina low, *Historical Archaeology*, 27, 3, 57–73.

Kwon, H. (n.d.) *Writing an International History from a Village Ethnography*. Online. Available www.lse.ac.uk/anthropology/events/Conferences/Pitch%20of%20Ethnography/Writing_an_International_History_from_a_Village_Ethnography.pdf (accessed 6 September 2013).

Kuppers, P. (2003) *Disability and Contemporary Performance: Bodies on Edge*, Abingdon: Routledge.

Larsen, N. (2000) Imperialism, colonialism, postcolonialism, in H. Schwarz and S. Ray (eds) *A Companion to Postcolonial Studies*, London: Blackwell.

Latour, B. (2010) *On the Modern Cult of the Factish Gods*, London: Duke University Press.

Lawson, A. (2006) Captain Silverspoons and His Missing Earring. Online. Available http://alanlawson.co.uk/creativewritingpage/captain-silverspoons/captain-silverspoons-and-his-missing-earring/#.U3x0mdJdWSo (accessed 21 May 2014).

Meekosha, H. (2011) Decolonising disability: thinking and acting globally, *Disability & Society*, 26, 6, 667–82.

Meskell, L. (2007) Falling walls and mending fences. Archaeological ethnography in the Limpopo, *Journal of Southern African Studies*, 33, 2, 383–400.

Orser, C.E. (1990) Archaeological approaches to new world plantation, *Archaeological Method and Theory*, 2, 111–54.

Pavlov-West, R. (2009) *Space in Theory: Kristeva, Foucault, Deleuze (Spatial Practices)*, Amsterdam: Rodopi Numb.

Pels, P. (1997) The anthropology of colonialism: culture, history, and the emergence of western governmentality, *Annual Review of Anthropology*, 26, 163–83.

Pinto, D. (2004) Indoctrinating the youth of post-war Spain: a discourse analysis of a Fascist civics textbook, *Discourse & Society*, 15, 5, 649–67.

Quayson, A. (2000) Postcolonial and postmodernism, in H. Schwarz and S. Ray (eds) *A Companion to Postcolonial Studies*, London: Blackwell.

Radune, R.A. (2005) *Pequot Plantation: The Story of an Early Colonial Settlement*, New York: Research in Time publications.

Roux, V. (2007) Ethnoarchaeology: a non-historical science of reference necessary for interpreting the past, *Journal of Archaeological Method and Theory*, 14, 2, 153–78.

Said, E. (1993) *Culture and Imperialism*, London: Vintage.

Sandhill, O. (2005) *Strengthening Inclusive Education by Applying Rights-based Approaches to Education Programming*, paper presented to ISEC 2005, University of Strathclyde.

Shields, R. (1997) *Ethnography in the Crowd. The Body, Sociality and Globalisation in Seoul.* Online. Available www.ualberta.ca/~rshields/f/focaal.html (accessed 6 September 2013).

Slee, R. (2001) Driven to the margins: disabled students, inclusive schooling and the politics of possibility, *Cambridge Journal of Education*, 13, 2, 385–97.

Strathern, M. (1991) *Partial Connections*, Oxford: Rowman and Littlefield.

Van der Veer, P.T. (1995) *Nation and Migration: The Politics of Space in the South Asian Diaspora*, Philadelphia: University of Pennsylvania Press.

Whitehead, N.L., Heckenberger, M.J. and Simon, G. (2010) Materializing the past among the Lokono (Arawak) of the Berbice River Guyna, *Anthropology*, 114: 87–127.

Williams, R. (1961) *The Long Revolution*, London: Chatt.

Žižek, S. (2008) *Organs without Bodies – Gilles Deleuze.* Online. Available www.lacan. com/zizisolation.html (accessed 1 September 2010).

Žižek, S. (2009) *In Defense of Lost Causes*, London: Verso.

12 Creative subjects?

Critically documenting art education and disability

Claire Penketh

This chapter explores the intersection between art education and disability in papers published in the *International Journal of Art and Design Education* (IJADE) over the last 30 years, offering a critical document of the range of social attitudes toward disability. It is an attempt to apply a disability studies perspective to the 'problem' of art education, and a continuation of my personal exploration of the meaning and role of art education for all learners. It also reflects my endeavour to support a call for an informed understanding of exclusionary processes inherent in specific curricular and pedagogical practices by examining beliefs and attitudes about disability through writing about art education (Moore and Slee, 2012).

In his chapter in the *Routledge Handbook of Disability Studies*, David Bolt asks if the study of culture can deepen our understanding of disability, and if the study of disability can therefore deepen our understanding of culture (Bolt, 2012). This interrelationship is discussed here in relation to the specific educational context of art education. In exploring the extent to which a study of art education can deepen our understanding of disability, I am also concerned with the extent to which a study of disability can deepen our understanding of art education. These ideas represent my continued interest in the distinctive contribution of art to education and exemplify the ways in which an interrogation of existing attitudes and practices can offer a useful starting point for transforming attitudes in education. The chapter explores changes in social attitudes by examining a range of discourses that have emerged over time, at the intersection of art education and disability. The aim is to explore the evolution of discourses at the intersection of art education and disability, the premise being that, in order to signal attitudinal change, it is essential to examine the attitudes that already exist.

In texts written to support current and future art educators, there appears to be a particular focus on provision for learners with so-called Special Educational Needs. Such texts are concerned with the identification of the particular needs of individuals, imparting knowledge about particular pedagogic interventions, categories of need, and a concern for 'including' pathologised learners. There is an unquestioning acceptance of their *special* status and the need for interventions to assure their inclusion in art education. Such textbooks appear to offer unproblematic representations of art education and how art teachers might or might not think about disability. For example, 'inclusive' strategies based around specific impairments are offered (Earle and Curry, 2005) that create problematic representations of disability and art education. Seemingly pragmatic solutions can promote assumptions about the role and nature of art education and appear to reinforce totalising attitudes toward disability. A concern with the pathologising tendencies of apparently pragmatic approaches offers another starting point for this chapter. The limitations of such approaches to teacher education based on 'the reductive reflex' that conflates inclusion in education with Special Educational Needs have been recognised (Moore and Slee, 2012: 230). The focus is on provision for the 'practical problem' of the disabled learner and future teachers are rarely challenged to consider the politics of disablement inherent in contemporary curricular, pedagogy, and assessment practices. The papers reviewed here from *IJADE*, therefore, relate to art education in a range of educational settings including mainstream and segregated provision, hospitals, prisons, and galleries. Such work, from a range of international perspectives, offers an opportunity to interrogate the ways in which disability has been conceptualised, over time, through writing about art education.

Art education, in this context, refers to education in the visual and tactile arts in compulsory education. Traditionally the lines have been drawn around visual arts education, although moves to incorporate contemporary practices have resulted in a more expansive range of approaches (e.g., video installations, performance art, and conceptual art pieces examining the use of text and ready-mades). An engagement with creative processes through art has been described as an essential educative practice and a number of authors over time have identified the importance of art practice and creativity to learning (Read, 1970; Brice-Heath, 2000; Eisner, 2002; Ruskin, 2007; Hickman, 2010). Knowledge and understanding of the art, craft, and design of others, sometimes described as contextual studies or visual studies, have also been included as a central aspect of the curriculum in the United Kingdom, Europe, and the United States.

Art education has traditionally been associated with the development of practical skills and control through fine art practice (Penketh, 2011), yet there is a recognition that education through art can be a powerful pedagogic tool, capable of transforming the lives of young people by enabling them to engage with significant ideas about their own cultural identities (Dash, 2005; Johnston, 2005). There are ongoing debates about the tensions between individual creative production and the requirement for the replication of specific skills. Arthur Hughes (1998) raised significant questions about the relevance of outmoded art practices that had little value or meaning to the lives of young people. More recently there have been moves to explore contemporary art and engage with art education as critical social practice, recognising the importance of art education to identity work. Atkinson and Dash have discussed the connections between art education with the potentially transformative nature of critical pedagogy advocating for 'art in education as a critical social practice' that 'has indirect but radical implications for implementing and renewing the systems within which teaching and learning take place' (Atkinson and Dash, 2005: xii).

Art practice is described by Julie Allan as an antidote to 'disciplinary regimes', offering opportunities for what she calls 'tactical defiance and resistance' (Allan, 2008: 86), yet art education is also subject to these regimes, with learners and educators defined by regulatory practices and subject to assessment processes that can lead to replication of a product rather than 'real' learning (Atkinson, 2001). There is potential for transformative critical practices in art education, and writers in the United States (Blandy, 1994; Derby, 2011; Wexler, 2011) have made connections between critical social practices associated with Disability Studies and art education, although such connections are less apparent in the United Kingdom. The present discussion of work intersecting art education and disability is therefore cognisant of the complex socio-political context of art education and the on-going struggle to maintain a significant and meaningful place for art in the school curriculum, particularly in the United Kingdom (Adams, 2013).

Exploring disability discourses in *IJADE*

IJADE is an international peer-reviewed journal with a particular focus on art and design education. First published in 1982, the journal is closely aligned to the work of the National Society for Education in Art and Design (NSEAD), an organisation established in the United Kingdom in 1944 to promote pedagogy in art and design. A study of papers published in the journal offers potential insight into discourses relating to the development of research in art and design education. I started reading *IJADE* while studying on a postgraduate teaching course in art and design in 1991 and am now one of the joint co-editors. There is therefore a strong autobiographical connection here: my own selection processes are implicated in the production/reproduction of particular discourses, so I must acknowledge a degree of reflexivity in the process of selection and analysis of papers (Rose, 2012: 197).

Fourteen papers were identified in my initial search, although it is important to note that other work may carry less explicit explorations of disability. The first article, 'The original art of mentally-handicapped people' (Timmerman, 1986), was published four years after the inaugural volume. The final article, 'Dyslexia and the studio: bridging the gap between theory and practice' by Alden and Pollock, was published in 2011. There have been over 900 papers published in the last 30 years and approximately 14 of these make an explicit reference to disability. Here, I am more concerned with the range and types of discourse in the papers identified than questions regarding underrepresentation of work about disability, although that too would be an appropriate line of enquiry.

To inform the theoretical framework of the chapter I draw on the work of Michel Foucault, particularly his interrogation of the effects of disciplinary power on the production and reproduction of knowledge (Foucault, 1991). His own working process has been described as an archeological one, creating and examining layers of knowledge (Foucault, 1980: 81–82). This 'lamination' is a compelling idea when considering discourses, created over time, in one particular journal. This tracing of Foucauldian 'systems of thought' examines the ways in which 'knowledge' about disability has been conveyed via explorations of art education, and the ways in which knowledge about art education has been conveyed via representations of disability. Foucault's exploration of discourse recognises that the formation of power/knowledge is relational. Power is not wielded from above but is part of the complex and complicit relationships between bodies, people or organisations (Foucault, 1991). Work published in a peer-reviewed journal, attached to the work of a learned society, constitutes a particular form of 'official knowledge', where sediments of professional and academic knowledge, set down over time, constitute a distillation of discourses that are therefore claimed as official knowledge. Foucault recognises that official knowledge forms occlude others. He states, 'Subjugated knowledges are thus those blocks of historical knowledge which were present but disguised within the body of functionalist and systematising theory and which criticism ... has been able to reveal' (Foucault, 1980: 81–82). Importantly, these official knowledge forms also act as instruments of normalisation, enabling the division of the pathological from the ideal. There is then a process of revelation in examining discourses that dominate and therefore subjugate others. In a journal whose focus is on art education, representations of disability can be read as a sub-text, harnessed to strengthen arguments for the essential nature of art education.

The 14 articles focus on art education, and representations of disability exist as a subtext. The 'systems of thought' exposed enable us to question the ways in which subtle and coercive forms of power have been exerted through a particular form of disciplinary knowledge. A central concern in a number of these publications is inclusion/exclusion in art education in school and gallery contexts, with some identifying projects designed to promote the inclusion of disabled learners (Corlett, 1994; Candlin, 2003; De Coster and Loots, 2004; Penketh, 2007). Hermon and Prentice (2003) promote the acknowledgement of difference and question forms of representation and identity formation. Their project is defined as 'boundary breaking' (Hermon and Prentice, 2003: 269), and offers the opportunity to challenge preconceptions about image and identity for learners who may experience stigma as a result of their *Special Education* status. The dominance of visual engagement as the normalising discourse in gallery and museum practices is challenged (Candlin, 2003), although tactile experience is still framed as a compensatory experience for those who are visually impaired. Although these papers recognise inequalities in the provision of art education and seek to address issues of access, they appear to do so from the 'veiled subject position' of the normate (Garland-Thomson, 1997: 8), confirming a distance between the 'expert' art educator and 'included' learner. Aims to include the Other can render us complicit in replicating the processes of Othering that we are trying to resist (Graham and Slee, 2008). However, this concern with bringing in the Other at least acknowledges a centre of practice that has previously excluded a range of learners. The main focus of the remaining discussion, therefore, lies with the ways in which art education is promoted through processes of normalisation that appear to be less conscious of an inherent disabling discourse.

Processes of normalisation

In *The Birth of the Clinic*, Foucault describes the dominance of ocularcentrism, where the medical discourse is authorised by the medical gaze, 'the eye that knows and decides, the eye that governs' (Foucault, 1976: 88). This knowledge form is authorised by professional knowledge and observation is connected with a kind of institutional knowing, a professional knowledge that exerts power. The role of observation is significant in the identification of difference as the observer is 'always receptive to the deviant'. In a number of the papers under discussion here, authors are observers of the Other and learners are recognised in terms of 'differences, variations, and anomalies' through their art practice and art products. There is power in the expert knowledge derived from these observations and this compares with the depiction of naive 'looking' in the learner's work (e.g., Dowling, 1994). Art practice becomes a process of surveillance and identification of difference and anomaly. The prioritisation of the professional gaze ensures that professional judgements dominate and this is reinforced by the 'faulty' observations of the learner.

Drawing practices in particular offer evidence of the ways in which normalising judgements are made about a person's ability to learn. The drawing becomes a site for pathology. Here there is a blurring between education and medical practices where drawings are subject to a 'normalising' aesthetic as well as a medical gaze. One paper, 'Drawing on the wrong side of the brain: an art teacher's case for recognising non-verbal learning disorders' (Warren, 2003), exemplifies this blurring of the boundaries between practice and diagnosis. The author argues for a greater recognition of this specific 'disorder', contending that art lessons could have 'a valuable diagnostic role, with observational work as a "window" into the right-brain' (Warren, 2003: 332). The pseudo-scientific foundation of this and a more recent paper exploring the experiences of students identified as dyslexic (Alden and Pollock, 2011) legitimises the definitions of the pathologised learner by reinforcing medical definitions of impairment. The value of art education appears to be enhanced by this pseudo-scientific, diagnostic value and it becomes complicit in a process of Othering. In this context the process is used effectively, although perhaps unconsciously, to reinforce our understanding of how and why art should be taught.

The disciplinary knowledge subject to exploration in the papers by Alden and Pollock, and Warren is implicated in the reading of both text and image. Photographs of learners and examples of artwork reinforce the 'truth' of what is presented in the text. For example, images of creative practice may provide evidence of creative growth and educability, but are also inscribed with the art teacher's specialist knowledge in defining learner pathology. Photographs and artwork can be described as socially produced, even where the practice appears to represent individual creative practice, since original artwork is repurposed to work with these authorised texts. Foucault suggests that in making some things visible, visuality may also act as a mask (Rose, 2012: 193). For example, in Dowling (1994), drawings by children identified as having 'moderate learning difficulties' are examined in order to understand developmental delay. 'Errors' in spatial representation are reproduced alongside photographs of Liverpool's Catholic cathedral (the building that they are aiming to represent in their drawings), producing a particularly convincing 'truth effect' and evidence of the learner pathology made evident through their drawing. This is also exemplified in photographs in Young (2008) and Taylor (2005), where access to art practice via the use of technology for 'supported learners' occludes their presence as creative practitioners. I discuss Taylor's paper as a specific example later in the chapter.

In other papers, learners' drawings exemplifying creative development are also reclaimed to signify learner pathology, and art education appears to have the potential for revealing the abnormal. One of the participants in Timmerman's study, 'Jaap', is described as 'a reticent and mildly retarded resident aged 45' (Timmerman, 1986: 120). Timmerman suggests that Jaap 'keeps himself occupied with various creative activities, working with the utmost concentration' (Timmerman, 1986: 120). With this textual translation it becomes impossible to view Jaap's drawings as anything other than the product of an impaired learner whose creativity, and therefore humanness, has been recognised by the interventions of the art educator. Although the 'meaning' in Jaap's work is unclear (since meaning is attributed by the reader and author), the work appears to have a degree of transparency, becoming a window into Jaap's creative potential. The inclusion of Jaap's 'authentic' creative product adds credibility to the author's account of the value of art education. Definitions of ability and disability are produced and reinforced by this process of 'discursive visuality'. The prints, produced by this 'middle-aged', 'reticent and mildly retarded' man, become implicated in the creation of our expectations of normalised ideas about image making. Similarly, the 'abnormal' drawings produced by children with 'learning difficulties', presented by Dowling, reinforce a normalised view of drawing development.

Creative practice is also examined as a compensatory mode of communication, as an emotional outlet, or for the development of coordination and skills. Here learners are reinforced as *disabled* by a particular need for creative practice, through art education, and the celebration of a universal need for art education is given particular credence by the creation of the disabled learner. Sagan (2009) examines art education and so-called mental ill health where art practice is recognised as a means of communication that might otherwise be denied. This is described as a kind of therapeutic release and a light to counterbalance narratives of misery and the dark places associated with mental ill health. Art practice is framed as a good for the 'sick' individual. This appears to contain art producer and practice in a 'closed loop', where therapeutic affect is limited to the producer and there is little consideration of the aesthetic significance of the work for others, or for any other educative value. Sagan offers two examples of student work, but there is little contextual information and the educative nature of this practice remains mysterious to the reader.

Paine (1997) explores the 'early obsessive drawings' of an individual identified as autistic, whose art practice is defined as offering a particular creative outlet for fear and anxiety. 'Obsessive drawing', as it is defined here, is offered as a means of communication that is pathologised as obsessive and compensatory for the other deficits that the child appears to exhibit. His art practice, now legitimised by his status as an adult and a practising artist, appeared unhealthy when associated with continuous autonomous production – early obsessive drawings sit beyond the control of the art teacher, and the art practices are considered excessive and therefore deviant. The imperative to include the Other in formalised educational processes may be construed here as a bid to authorise and lay claim to art practices that exist outside of the regulatory space of compulsory mainstream schooling.

Acts of erasure

Most of the papers under consideration are implicated in processes of normalisation where art education for the disabled learner becomes a site for identification of difference, support, compensation, and/or remediation. I argue here that this fact positions the work in the domain of a Special Educational Needs discourse that appears to subjugate the potential for a critical discussion of disability. My main argument is that the special education discourse in *IJADE* evidences a relational dimension or 'discursive formation' (Rose, 2012: 191). In aiming to elevate issues of access and inclusion to art education, both subjects (disabled learner and art education) are represented as a series of practical and technical problems to be solved. Importantly, the potential of both learner and subject appears to be diminished by the dominance of this discourse. The final section of this chapter offers a more detailed exploration of the ways in which a focus on support, working as a normalising discourse, erases the disabled learner and her or his practice. I therefore return to the paper by Taylor (2005), 'Access and support in the development of a visual language: arts education and disabled students'.

Taylor focuses on the experiences of three learners, Jo, Sam, and Anthony, and outlines the use of enablers and the deployment of technology to support the art production of disabled students in post 16 education. Taylor suggests that practical assistance in the form of the use of enablers and ICT can provide 'seamless access to the visual arts for disabled students' in order to 'express their particular experiences of the human condition' (Taylor, 2005: 325). A photograph showing 'Jo using an interactive whiteboard' has a specific focus on the means of production and of Jo 'using' rather than making or creating a piece of art work. The second image is of Anthony, working with an enabler. The assistant is in the foreground manipulating a piece of chicken wire and Anthony is in the background observing or directing. Both students are presented as supported learners, and there is little interest in what or why they are aiming to produce. The third student, Sam, only exists via a description of her reliance on technology. Taylor explains:

> The production of her art work is heavily reliant on digital and lens-based media with the addition of mark making produced with traditional materials that can be further manipulated digitally.
>
> (Taylor, 2005: 330)

An alternative representation could have described Sam as *specialising* in the use of digital technology. There are no photographs of Sam, who is therefore invisible as well as voiceless. Her apparent inability to communicate is presented as a further barrier to her creative engagement, and we are informed that communication can be 'extremely time consuming and open to misinterpretation if the enabler is not entirely familiar with the student' (Taylor, 2005: 330). Although Taylor emphasises the use of ICT in enabling art production, there is no recognition of Sam's work and she is framed as a series of technical problems to be overcome. What does she make? Why does she make it? What does it look or feel like? What does it mean? Sam's work and her identity as a creative practitioner are erased. Taylor writes, 'Sam and many other disabled students are empowered by the knowledge that, with technological and enabling support, the realisation of creative ideas is not blighted or confined by physical limitations' (Taylor, 2005: 330), yet this representation of Sam impacts on our perception of her ability to engage with creative practice.

Of further interest to me here is the representation of art education and the focus on the technologies of physical production. This limited and limiting representation of disability reinforces a narrow view of art education as a subject concerned with technical production, rather than the conceptualisation and realisation of creative practice. The negation of the creative subjects, Jo, Sam, and Anthony, therefore conveys a diminished form of art education.

Conclusion

In this chapter I examine a range of texts that explores art education and disability. In so doing, I aim to raise consciousness about the ways in which writing about art education have reflected and reproduced particular ideas about disability, and recognise that in many cases this has resulted in the reinforcement of the epistemology of special education (Moore and Slee, 2012). Although Atkinson and Dash (2005) advocate for art education, as a critical and social practice, that creates possibilities for 'the critique of social systems', there appears to be a greater emphasis on the social systems that relate more directly to race, class, and gender, and it is possible to question whether there is an avoidance of criticality in work relating to disability (Bolt, 2012). The intersection between art education and disability in *IJADE* offers the potential to prioritise the voice of the disabled practitioner, the disabled art educator, or the transgressive and transformative potential of disability arts. I suggest that art educators could find a useful exemplification of critical and social practice if they looked beyond the boundaries of Special Educational Needs and into the politics of disablement.

Of significance for the present book is the ways in which attitudes can change, informed by and informing political and social context. It is unsurprising that some language used in the early papers would now be deemed unacceptable and it is perhaps heartening to reflect on the changes in the representation of disability in this respect. However, we must still question more recent work in *IJADE* that represents disabled people as abnormal, deficient, and in particular need of the 'special' gifts that an art education can bestow. Of greatest importance, perhaps, is the need to make future art educators aware that identifying the needs of the disabled learner as special is only one (fundamentally flawed) way of conceptualising learning in and through the arts, and that this is problematic for learner and teacher. If we recognise the value of art education for the development of learner identity through practical and creative expression, then it is vital that we do so from an informed perspective. This implies an understanding of critical disability studies by art educators and an application to their research and pedagogic practice.

References

Adams, J. (2013) Editorial: the English baccalaureate: a new philistinism? *International Journal of Art and Design Education*, 32, 1, 2–5.

Alden, S. and Pollock, V.L. (2011) Dyslexia and the studio: bridging the gap between theory and practice, *International Journal of Art and Design Education*, 30, 1, 81–89.

Allan, J. (2008) *Rethinking Inclusive Education – The Philosophers of Difference in Practice*, Dordrecht: Springer.

Atkinson, D. (2001) Assessment in educational practice: forming pedagogised identities in the art curriculum, *The International Journal of Art and Design Education*, 20, 1, 96–108.

Atkinson, D. and Dash, P. (2005) *Social and Critical Practices in Art Education*, Stoke on Trent: Trentham.

Blandy, D. (1994) Assuming responsibility: disability rights and the preparation of art, *Educators Studies in Art Education*, 35, 3, 179–187.

Bolt, D. (2012) Social encounters, cultural representation and critical avoidance, in N. Watson, A. Roulstone, and C. Thomas (eds) *Routledge Handbook of Disability Studies*, London: Routledge.

Brice Heath, S. (2000) Seeing our way into learning, *Cambridge Journal of Education*, 30, 1, 121–32.

Candlin, F. (2003) Blindness, art and exclusion in museums and galleries, *International Journal of Art and Design Education*, 22, 1, 100–10.

Corlett, S. (1994) Students with disabilities on fine art degrees, *Journal of Art and Design Education*, 13, 3, 267–73.

Dash, P. (2005) Culutural demarcation, the African diaspora and art education, in D. Atkinson and P. Dash (eds) *Social and Critical Practices in Art Education*, Stoke on Trent: Trentham.

De Coster, K. and Loots, G. (2004) Somewhere in between touch and vision: in search of a meaningful art education for blind individuals, *International Journal of Art and Design Education*, 23, 3, 326–34.

Derby, J. (2011) Disability studies and art education, *Studies in Art Education: A Journal of Issues and Research*, 52, 2, 94–111.

Dowling, S. (1994) Children's early drawing development and its links with special teaching abilities, *Journal of Art and Design Education*, 13, 3, 251–66.

Earle, K. and Curry, G. (2005) *Meeting SEN in the Curriculum: Art*, London: David Fulton.

Eisner, E. (2002) *The Arts and the Creation of Mind*, Yale: University Press.

Foucault, M. (1976) *The Birth of the Clinic*, London: Tavistock.

Foucault, M. (1980) *Power/Knowledge: Selected Interviews and Other Writings 1972–1977*, New York: Pantheon.

Foucault, M. (1991) *Discipline and Punish – The Birth of the Prison*, London: Penguin.

Garland-Thomson, R. (1997) *Extraordinary Bodies: Figuring Physical Disability in American Culture and Literature*, New York: Columbia University Press.

Graham, L. and Slee, R. (2008) An illusory interiority: interrogating the discourse/s of inclusion, *Educational Philosophy and Theory*, 40, 2, 277–92.

Hermon, A. and Prentice, R. (2003) Positively different: art and design in special education, *International Journal of Art and Design Education*, 22, 3, 268–80.

Hickman, R. (2010) *Why We Make Art and Why It Is Taught*, Bristol: Intellect.

Hughes, A. (1998) Reconceptualising the art curriculum, *Journal of Art and Design Education*, 17, 1, 41–49.

Johnston, J. (2005) Art in contentious spaces, in D. Atkinson and P. Dash (eds) *Social and Critical Practices in Art Education*, Stoke on Trent: Trentham.

Moore, M. and Slee, R. (2012) Disability studies, inclusive education and exclusion, in N. Watson, A. Roulstone, and C. Thomas (eds) *Routledge Handbook of Disability Studies*, London: Routledge.

Paine, S. (1997) Early obsessive drawings and personal development, *Journal of Art and Design Education*, 16, 2, 147–55.

Penketh, C. (2011) *A Clumsy Encounter: Dyspraxia and Drawing*, Rotterdam: Sense.

Penketh, C. (2007) Supporting pupils with dyspraxia in the visual arts: does drawing from observation function as an official and discriminatory discourse? *International Journal of Art and Design Education*, 26, 2, 144–154.

Read, H. (1970) *Education through Art*, London: Faber and Faber.

Rose, G. (2012) *Visual Methodologies*, London: Sage.

Ruskin, J. (2007) *The Elements of Drawing*, London: A. and C. Black.

Sagan, O. (2009) Open disclosures: learning, creativity and the passage of mental (ill) health, *International Journal of Art and Design Education*, 28, 1, 107–16.

Taylor, M. (2005) Access and support in the development of visual language: arts education and disabled students, *International Journal of Art and Design Education*, 24, 3, 325–33.

Timmerman, M. (1986) The original art of mentally-handicapped people, *Journal of Art and Design Education*, 5, 1–2, 111–23.

Warren, R. (2003) Drawing on the wrong side of the brain: an art teacher's case for recognising – NLD, *International Journal of Art and Design Education*, 22, 3, 325–34.

Wexler, A. (2011) *Art and Disability: The Social and Political Struggles Facing Education*, Basingstoke: Palgrave MacMillan.

Young, G. (2008) Autonomy and artistic expression for adult learners with disabilities, *International Journal of Art and Design Education*, 27, 2, 116–23.

13 Dysrationalia

An institutional learning disability?

Owen Barden

Contemporaneously with the publication of Lennard Davis's *Enforcing Normalcy* in 1995, Keith Stanovich, an eminent Canadian psychologist, was questioning the conceptual foundations of learning disabilities. To illustrate his critique he invented a new learning disability that he called dysrationalia (Stanovich, 1993). Around the same time, Peter Senge's seminal management book *The Fifth Discipline* was encouraging people to credit organisations with the ability to learn and even to have learning disabilities (Senge, 1990). True to the interdisciplinary ethos of disability studies, in this chapter I draw on current and historical perspectives from discourses including philosophy, critical and cognitive psychology, and organisation management to ask if dysrationalia can help to explain social attitudes toward disability as they occur within organisations.

Dysrationalia

Stanovich introduced the concept of *dysrationalia* in 1993. As a cognitive psychologist and long-term critic of the 'selective deficit' models often used to define specific learning disabilities, he was making a point about the way such disabilities are conceptualised and operationalised in psychological discourse. The logic is that specific learning difficulties are defined by identifying an apparent discrepancy between a person's level of achievement in a specific skill domain and her or his overall intelligence as measured by an IQ test; that to do this, psychologists must dissociate specific cognitive skills from intelligence; that they are able to do this because of the narrowness of the cognitive domains tapped by IQ tests; and that, therefore, to 'find' a new specific learning disability, all we need do is choose a cognitive domain outside those tapped by IQ tests, measure it, and then find an apparent discrepancy between some people's achievements in that domain and their intelligence as measured by an IQ test. Dyslexia, for example, is 'found' when a psychologist establishes a statistically significant discrepancy between a person's literacy attainments and her or his IQ score.

Stanovich extended the logic of diagnosis to invent a new specific learning difficulty, *dysrationalia*. Aping the format used for existing specific learning difficulties, he defined dysrationalia as an enduring disposition characterised by:

The inability to think and behave rationally despite adequate intelligence. It is a general term that refers to a heterogeneous group of disorders manifested by significant difficulties in belief formation, in the assessment of belief consistency, and/or in the determination of action to achieve one's goals. Although dysrationalia may occur concomitantly with other handicapping conditions (e.g. sensory impairment), it is not the result of those conditions. The key diagnostic criterion for dysrationalia is a level of rationality, as demonstrated in thinking and behaviour, that is significantly below the level of the individual's intellectual capacity (as determined by an individually administered IQ test).

(Stanovich, 1993: 503)

Stanovich gave some helpful examples to illustrate apparent real-life cases of dysrationalia. These included a survey on the paranormal beliefs of members of a Mensa club in Canada. Mensa members must evidence high IQs, yet in this Canadian branch 56 per cent reported believing in the existence of extraterrestrial visitors and 44 per cent reported believing in astrology: beliefs for which 'there is no valid evidence' (Stanovich, 1993: 503). His point was that adequate or even high IQ does not inoculate people against 'significant difficulties in belief formation', because the intelligent people in these examples readily formed and maintained irrational beliefs (i.e., beliefs that lack any convincing evidence base).

Rationality

The concept of dysrationalia explicitly relies on the concept of rationality. Rationality, it has been argued, was the central idea of the Enlightenment (Venn, 1984). Philosophers' Enlightenment conception of rationality was for human beings to rely on their own structured processes of thinking, judgement, and reasoning to decide what is right and true, and how to act. Philosophy's association with science meant that, from the seventeenth century, many Western philosophers and scientists assumed that people are inherently rational beings, choosing the actions that best fit their self-determined, reasoned goals. This *'homo rationalis'* (Venn, 1984: 119) attitude is still influential in cognitive and developmental psychology today (Gergely et al., 2002).

It could be argued that this normative assumption of instrumental rationality is inherently disabling, laying the foundations for psychology's historical obsession with deviance, and attitudes geared toward treatment and control (Goodley, 2012). In addition, the Industrial Revolution's preoccupation with amplifying the powers and maximising the utility of the human body in order to meet the efficiency demands of the military and the economic mode of production (Morgan, 2006) led to ideologies of oppression and the marginalisation of people with impairments (Barnes and Mercer, 2003). As the Industrial Revolution progressed, the concept of rationality was applied to organisations and companies as they sought to maximise profits. This gave rise to bureaucracy and 'scientific' management styles that characterised organisations as machines and viewed the human element within them as a technical problem that needed to be controlled, so that people would fit the machine and the machine would work as efficiently as possible. People with impairments were viewed less favourably because they did not fit the machine well. Moreover, the new system of universal schooling, designed to create workers for the industrial economy, helped instrumental rationality become associated with attitudes of domination, oppression, discrimination, and totalitarianism in education (Han, 2002).

One consequence of these prejudices is the troubled relationship between psychology and disability (Goodley, 2012). However, rather than perpetuating antagonism, here I follow the call to try and make allies of these disciplines (Goodley and Lawthom, 2006). I discuss some evidence from psychology that may help explain personal and organisational responses to disability, appropriating and repurposing *dysrationalia* to give insights into both rationality and social attitudes toward disability.

Stanovich views rational thinking as a disposition, a cognitive style related to an individual's processes of belief formation and decision making. This is an instrumental view of rationality characterised by a means-end philosophy – in order to be rational, people must choose actions based on sound reasons to get what they want. He distinguishes three components of rational thinking: belief formation, belief consistency, and action determination (Stanovich, 1993). Belief formation concerns the way information about the world fixes beliefs. Belief consistency refers to a process by which people monitor how well their beliefs match their aims and desires. Action determination concerns processes by which people use their beliefs about the world to decide on which actions to take in order to satisfy their desires. Thus, for people to think and act rationally, they must choose actions that demonstrate logical consistency with their beliefs and desires. This outline is expanded by seven requirements of the rational thinking disposition:

1   Choice of action is optimal given goals and beliefs;
2   Collecting information before making up one's mind;
3   Seeking various points of view before coming to a conclusion;
4   Calibrating the degree of strength of one's opinion to the degree of evidence available;
5   Thinking about consequences before taking action;
6   Explicitly weighing the positives and negatives of a situation;
7   Seeking nuance and avoiding absolutism.

(Stanovich et al., 2011: 796)

In summary, to be rational, a person must have well-calibrated beliefs – beliefs that are commensurate with the available evidence (epistemic rationality) – and must act appropriately on those beliefs to achieve her or his goals (instrumental rationality). However, it has been noted that 'Modelling of the external world by beliefs … may become so poor that we want to call it irrational' (Stanovich, 1993: 504). In a similar vein, it has been observed that 'human judgement is overly influenced by vivid but unrepresentative personal and case evidence and under-influenced by more representative and diagnostic, but pallid, statistical evidence'

(Stanovich and West, 2000: 647). I suggest that the vivid, largely negative, stereotypical mental representations non-disabled people tend to hold of disabled people (Bolt, 2012) are thus likely to have exaggerated influence on modelling of the world and hence belief formation and attitudes of people and the organisations they constitute. This produces irrational behaviour and prejudicial attitudes when confronted with disability and disabled people: not collecting sufficient information about disability and disabled people before making up minds; not seeking the various views of disabled and non-disabled people sufficiently; not calibrating opinions to the evidence available; not thinking through consequences fully before taking action; not explicitly weighing positives and negatives of situations before acting; not seeking nuance and so tending to absolutism.

Dysrationality

So to be dysrational means to have an inability to think and act rationally despite adequate intelligence. People tend to think they are behaving rationally (i.e., logically and in accordance with their own best interests), yet some psychologists argue that, contrary to the assumption that humans are rational beings, people's thoughts and actions are often systematically irrational. That is to say, their actions are not logical or do not serve their own best interests (Kahneman and Tversky, 1984; Kahneman, 2011). Why might this be so? In this discussion I set aside the methodological issues inherent in cognitive psychology's laboratory interpretations of rationality in experiment participants (Stanovich and West, 2000) and instead focus on insights from that field on how people think, and how their thinking determines their actions.

When not measuring, classifying, and treating people they deem to be abnormal for one reason or another, psychologists try to understand how people think. Cognitive psychologists talk of two kinds of thinking, Type 1 (T1) and Type 2 (T2). T1 thinking is held to be a kind of default setting. It is automatic and autonomous: a continuous, low effort response to the information arriving from the senses. It is the kind of thinking many of us do without realising we are thinking, such as when we interpret the emotions on someone's face. This is sometimes called *fast thinking* because it is quick and virtually effortless (Kahneman, 2011). In contrast, T2 thinking involves deliberate analysis, such as when we try to do long division in our heads; it requires a conscious decision to reflect on information, is effortful, and thus called *slow thinking* (Kahneman, 2011).

In the 1970s, social scientists broadly accepted two ideas about human nature: first, that people are generally rational, and their thinking is normally sound; second, that emotions such as fear, affection, and hatred explain most of the occasions on which people depart from rationality (Kahneman, 2011). Since then, a field known within the domain of psychology as *heuristics and biases* has emerged. This field examines the role of knowledge bases on rationality. That is to say, the field is concerned with the way the autonomous mind retrieves overlearned knowledge derived from experience and how this knowledge impinges on rationality. Evidence from cognitive studies of decision making in this field suggests that it is *not* simply 'corruption' of thought by emotion that explains most instances of irrationality: instead, flaws in the design of the machinery of cognition predispose people to irrational thought.

Cognitive psychologists argue that fast T1 thinking (which is impressionistic, rapid, and hence error-prone) is our default setting. Yet rational thinking demands both fast T1 and slow T2: the analytic mind must consciously reason, overruling the intuitive, impulsive one. Unfortunately, people tend not to engage T2 (i.e., 'the lazy controller') *because* it is slow and effortful. This inherent bias toward fast, low-effort thinking and our aversion to analysis means that people tend to overgeneralise from past experience, and tend not to modify their beliefs in the face of new evidence or information, so that their attitudes and actions frequently lack a rational basis.

For example, it has been noted how the *availability heuristic* introduces bias in our thinking according to how readily examples come to mind: examples that are particularly dramatic, sensational, or personal will lead us to overestimate the frequency of particular events or the significance of particular issues (Kahneman, 2011). This bias toward the vivid yet unrepresentative may help to explain irrational social attitudes toward disability. Accordingly, persistent sensationalist, derogatory reporting of disability benefit fraud and the pejorative language used in British tabloid newspapers leads people to overestimate the scale of disability benefit fraud tenfold – and this has in turn been linked to a society-wide hardening of attitudes and even increased disability hate crime (Briant et al., 2011).

Heuristics and biases thus offer one explanation for the frequent failure of slow T2 to override fast T1 and enable us to think rationally. In addition, although emotion alone cannot explain why people depart from rationality, every stimulus is automatically held to generate an affective evaluation of its 'goodness' or 'badness' (Kahneman and Frederickson, 2002). In other words, all of our thinking is mediated by emotional associations, which may be conscious or unconscious. T1 thinking helps people regulate their behaviour in accordance with their emotions and will sometimes prompt a fast, rational response, such as to move away from a frightening and dangerous animal. However, there will be occasions where we need to override our emotional responses and think slowly in order to think and act rationally. We might, for instance, need to override the emotion of disgust if we needed to take an unpleasant-tasting medicine in order to recover our health. This is where T2 thinking comes in. In order to generate the rational response, it is argued that T2 thinking must recognise the bias caused by emotional association and correct the initial emotional response generated in T1 thinking through intentional reasoning and cognitive simulation of a 'better' (i.e., more rational) response in relation to the individual's beliefs, desires, and goals. A further potential source of irrationality, then, is the failure of T2 thinking to overcome the emotional responses generated automatically in T1 thinking.

What are the emotions, stereotypes, and representations associated with disability and disabled people that might dominate and disrupt the initial reactions to impairment? Not untypically, fear, pity, and disgust have been highlighted (Hughes, 2012). It seems reasonable to suggest that negative emotions and their overlearned associations, mediated in part by society and culture (Powell and Gilbert, 2008), help form the foundations for stigma (Goffman, 1963; Bolt, 2012) and the thinking disposition known as prejudice: 'irrational, pervasive and enduring sentiment' (Katz, 1991: 127) that results in hostility toward, and avoidance of, minority groups. This is borne out in the evidence from cognitive psychology discussed here.

It seems clear that emotion plays a significant role in people's reasoning, and that the rationalist attempt to separate intellect and emotion is misguided (Gabriel and Griffiths, 2002). Human judgement and hence attitudes are overly influenced by easily recalled, vivid representations. There is 'probably as much irrationality in our feelings … as there is in our choice of actions' and 'specific features of problem content, and their semantic associations, constitute the dominant influence on thought' with the result that 'beliefs which have served us well are not lightly abandoned' (Stanovich and West, 2000: 655, 661). Rationality is further hampered by our tendency to contextualise a problem with as much prior knowledge as possible, to make assumptions and then reason from those assumptions, and to engage in narrative modes of thought that result in failure to engage in the cognitive abstraction necessary to arrive at a rational response. In other words, people tend to rely on their existing beliefs and on incomplete, invalid or oversimplified representations when faced with difficult issues. These insights from cognitive psychology overlap strikingly with the claim from a disability studies perspective that when one person has a visible impairment, it tends to dominate another's processing of perceptions, to have a disruptive influence on her or his initial reactions (Garland-Thomson, 1997; Bolt, 2012).

Researchers in heuristics and biases have repeatedly demonstrated that people, regardless of intelligence, habitually violate the precepts of rationality: they tend toward confirmation bias, they do not test hypotheses thoroughly, they do not accurately calibrate their beliefs to the evidence available, and they over-project their own opinions onto others (Stanovich et al., 2011). Individual differences in rationality may be partially attributable to variations in intelligence, but high intelligence alone does not inoculate against irrationality – as in the case of the Canadian Mensa members. The claim is that many different studies involving thousands of subjects have indicated that measures of intelligence display only moderate to weak or near-zero correlations with thinking dispositions associated with rational thought (Stanovich et al., 2011: 792). So it seems that many if not most people are predisposed to dysrationalia. But how can the same be said of organisations?

The discussion of individual cognition and personal instances of dysrationalia is necessary to develop an understanding of the concept and how it might come about. But the title of this chapter asks whether dysrationalia might be more helpfully thought of as an *organisational* learning disability, rather than an individual one. In other words, can organisations show inability to act rationally despite adequate intelligence? It is perhaps important to consider what is meant by an *organisation* before discussing whether or not organisations can have a learning disability. Organisations are made up of people engaged in a shared endeavour, assets and resources, and physical presence, yet are somehow more than the sum of these parts: we cannot point to something and say 'that is an organisation' (Stacey, 2003). This ineffability has produced a tendency to invoke metaphors to describe organisations. As noted, from the time of the Industrial Revolution, and closely tied to the idea of instrumental rationality, one enduring metaphor has been that of the organisation-as-machine. Another enduring image is that of organisation-as-brain (Morgan, 2006). Like brains, organisations process vast amounts of information in order to monitor internal processes and the outside world, and to make decisions; tasks are distributed and specialised but the whole works together toward common goals; those goals are related to the beliefs and values of the organisation; there are complex patterns and interactions between the interdependent parts that make it self-organising.

If we accept the brain metaphor, it follows that we accept that organisations can be intelligent and can learn, because learning and intelligence are defining characteristics of brains. Since the early 1990s, a considerable literature has emerged that deals with organisational intelligence and learning. Seminal here was Senge's *The Fifth Discipline*, which introduced the concept of the learning organisation. Regrettably, he does not offer a concrete definition of a learning organisation (Örtenblad, 2007), but instead, in somewhat evangelical tones, describes their characteristics in various ways throughout the book:

> A learning organisation is one where people continually expand their capacity to create the results they truly desire, where new and expansive patterns of thinking are nurtured, where collective aspiration is set free, and where people are continually learning how to learn together.
>
> (Senge, 1990: 3)

This description is particularly salient to my discussion. First, the final clause indicates that it is not organisations *per se* that learn (how could they if they are not 'things'?) but the people within them who learn together. Second, we can detect a strongly instrumental-rationalist subtext in the idea of continually expanding people's capacity to create the results they desire. Third, in the light of the preceding discussion, we can see a potential problem. In a learning organisation *new and expansive patterns of thinking are nurtured* – but hardly anyone is predisposed toward new and expansive patterns of thinking. As we have seen, people tend to stick to beliefs and thinking dispositions they already have, even when these are faulty, incomplete, biased or counterproductive. To an extent, Senge anticipated this, entitling the second chapter of the book 'Does your organisation have a learning difficulty?' (Senge, 1990). He argued that it was no accident that most organisations learned poorly 'despite the best efforts of bright, committed people' (Senge, 1990: 18) and therefore failed to act rationally despite the adequate collective intelligence of the people working there.

Key here is the concept of mental models. Mental models are one of the five 'disciplines' or dimensions Senge argues organisations need to master in order to learn. He describes mental models as deeply ingrained images, assumptions, and stories of how the world works, which limit us to familiar ways of thinking and acting. He argues that they are 'active' in that they not only determine how we perceive the world but also shape how we act, quoting another luminary, Chris Argyris of Harvard Business School:

> Although people do not [always] behave congruently with their espoused theories [what they say], they do behave congruently with their theories in use [their mental models].
>
> (Argyris, 1982 cited in Senge, 1990: 175)

The claim here is derived from cognitive psychology: that people model the world according to their beliefs, beliefs that often lack epistemic rationality – they do not accurately represent what is true – because they are overly influenced by vivid images and representations, and by unrepresentative prior experience (Stanovich and West, 2000). It follows that if people within organisations have negative, stereotypical images of disability then their mental models will be flawed. These flawed mental models will shape action in ways that are likely to be detrimental to disabled people. For example, common stereotypes include disabled people being sinister, deviant, or simply incapable (Barnes, 1992). Moreover, because people are reluctant to reject ideas that have served them well, non-disabled people seem doubly unlikely to update their mental models when they encounter people who are disabled.

As in the literature from psychology and disability studies, Senge highlights the role of emotion in regulating people's thinking and behaviour. Embarrassment, another emotion commonly associated with disability and impairment, is mentioned repeatedly as a response that overrides rational action. He notes how organisations from school onwards teach us to hide appearing uncertain or ignorant to protect ourselves from the embarrassment and ridicule of making mistakes in front of our peers and authority figures; how embarrassment frequently blocks new understandings and prevents people from learning; how people revert to 'defensive routines' that include avoiding raising difficult issues or significant disagreements when embarrassment looms or when they fear exposing invalid reasoning: 'When was the last time someone was rewarded in your organisation for raising difficult questions about the company's current policies rather than solving urgent problems?'(Senge, 1990: 249, 25). He argues that one consequence of inaccurate mental models, irrational, emotional responses and defensive routines is that teamwork breaks down as people fail to confront complex issues that may be embarrassing or threatening, senior members in the management hierarchy 'squelch' disagreement, and people avoid stating serious reservations and disagreements in order to maintain the appearance of a cohesive team (Senge, 1990: 24). In doing so, the team fails to examine the issue in a way that could result in everybody learning from each other, there is a lack of intentional reasoning, and hence the organisation fails to learn. In other words, poor epistemic rationality resulting from inaccurate mental models is compounded by people breaking the strictures of instrumental rationality as their reason is overridden by their emotions and they avoid collectively engaging with a complex, uncomfortable problem. As a result, the organisation fails to learn despite its members having adequate intelligence and capacity to learn. The organisation has dysrationalia.

Changing social attitudes

Having diagnosed pandemic dysrationalia, with most organisations learning poorly, I must conclude by considering the curative prescription. How might we foster more rational social attitudes toward disability in organisations? Perhaps surprisingly, there is something of a convergence of opinion here. Critiques of economic, instrumental rationality, insights from cognitive and critical psychology, exhortations from the management literature, and the voices of disabled people seem to point in the same overall direction: reflection and dialogue aimed at confronting inaccurate beliefs and irrational attitudes. First, the shift to a post-industrial, post-modernity epoch suggests that the materialist, instrumentally rationalist view of organisations is outmoded, and more attention needs to be paid to the social and ethical dimensions of work and 'progress' (Hinchcliff, 2006; White, 2006; White, 2013). Second, the suggestion from critical psychology for changing social attitudes toward disability is to shift the focus of attention from the individual to the collective (Venn, 1984), which means working alongside people in a community of inquiry in order to generate social change (Goodley and Lawthom, 2006).

Collective inquiry into uncomfortable issues, however, is something people tend to avoid, although some have argued that it is vital in any learning organisation (Senge, 1990; Gabriel and Griffiths, 2002; Smith and Sharma, 2002; Stacey, 2003). It is necessary to unearth and reflect on mental models in order to clarify assumptions, discover contradictions, and develop strategies to close the gap between the models and reality. This is termed *metanoia*: a shift of mind (Senge, 1990: 13). In the language of cognitive psychology, overlearned negative emotional and semantic associations must be unlearned through rational thought, or at least suspended to enable T2 thinking to recalibrate the automatic operations of T1 thinking. Attitudinal barriers need to be confronted so that knowledge about disability develops informed understanding of disability, stereotypes are challenged, and discrimination eliminated. Group discussion appears to increase rationality, and people can suspend their biases and think rationally when instructed how to do so (Stanovich and West, 2000; Kahneman, 2011).

Encouraging employees to be open about their attitudes and emotions and how they influence their thinking might raise the spectre of programmes that seek to elicit 'correct' emotional responses (Gabriel and Griffiths, 2002) to disability. But here an alternative conception of rationality, one that I have not yet discussed, may come into play. Jürgen Habermas, whose philosophy was shaped by childhood responses to his own disability as well as doubts over instrumental rationality (Clifford, 2012), argued for what he called *communicative rationality* (Han, 2002). Habermas felt that the cognitive interpretation of rationality obscured the role of intersubjectivity and dialogue in reasoning, with 'truth' not predetermined but arrived at through 'the force of the better argument' (Han,

2002: 152). The goal of communicative rationality is thus democratic and inclusive (Clifford, 2012): to arrive at mutual understanding and trust, not to reach instrumental goals. It focuses on establishing new, consensual social norms since social norms provide important motivation for action that is irreducible to instrumental or strategic rationality (Moon, 2006). Habermas observes that the collective efforts and sacrifices of sociopolitical movements must embody the principles and contextual application of rational thought in order to persuade others of the validity of their claims and determine action (Warnke, 2006: 133). The Disability Rights movement, therefore, has the role of 'making the better argument' and hence moving organisations toward rational, informed understanding of disability. For their part, organisations must listen and reason, then make decisions based on the weight of the evidence. Employees are not manipulated into responding 'correctly' to the 'problem' of disability but instead to fulfil the requirements of rational thinking (Stanovich et al., 2011): collecting information before making up one's mind; seeking various points of view before coming to a conclusion; calibrating the degree of strength of one's opinion to the degree of evidence available; thinking about consequences before taking action; explicitly weighing the positives and negatives; seeking nuance and avoiding absolutism; choosing optimal actions given goals and beliefs.

References

Barnes, C. (1992) Disabling imagery and the media: an exploration of the principles for media representations of disabled people. *British Council of Organisations of Disabled People*. Online. Available http://disability-studies.leeds.ac.uk/files/library/Barnes-disabling-imagery. pdf (accessed 30 October, 2013).

Barnes, C. and Mercer, G. (2003) *Disability*, Cambridge: Polity.

Bolt, D. (2012) Social encounters, cultural representation and critical avoidance, in N. Watson, A. Roulstone, and C. Thomas (eds) *Routledge Handbook of Disability Studies*, London: Routledge.

Briant, E., Watson, N., and Philo, G. (2011) Bad news for disabled people: how the newspapers are reporting disability. Online. Available http://eprints.gla.ac.uk/57499 (accessed 30 October, 2013).

Clifford, S. (2012) Making disability public in deliberative democracy, *Contemporary Political Theory*, 11, 211–28.

Davis, L.J. (1995) *Enforcing Normalcy: Disability, Deafness and the Body*, London: Verso.

Gabriel, Y. and Griffiths, D.S. (2002) Emotion, learning and organizing, *The Learning Organization*, 9, 5, 214–21.

Garland-Thomson, R. (1997) *Extraordinary Bodies: Figuring Physical Disability in American Culture and Literature*, New York: Columbia University Press.

Gergely, G., Bekkering, H., and Király, I. (2002) Rational imitation in preverbal infants, *Nature*, 415, 6873, 755.

Goffman, E. (1963) *Stigma: Notes on the Management of Spoiled Identity*, Middlesex: Penguin.

Goodley, D. (2012) The psychology of disability, in N. Watson, A. Roulstone, and C. Thomas (eds) *Routledge Handbook of Disability Studies*, Routledge: London.

Goodley, D. and Lawthom, R. (2006) Disability studies and psychology: new allies? In D. Goodley and R. Lawthom (eds) *Disability and Psychology*, Basingstoke: Palgrave.

Han, G. (2002) An educational interpretation of Jürgen Habermas's Communicative Rationality, *Asia Pacific Education Review*, 3, 2, 149–59.

Hinchcliff, J. (2006) The future of the university: some ethico-epistemological explorations, *On the Horizon*, 14, 2, 77–83.

Hughes, B. (2012) Fear, pity and disgust: emotions and the non-disabled imaginary, in N. Watson, A. Roulstone, and C. Thomas (eds) *Routledge Handbook of Disability Studies*, Routledge: London.

Kahneman, D. (2011) *Thinking, Fast and Slow*, London: Penguin.

Kahneman, D. and Tversky, A. (1984) Choices, values and frames, *American Psychologist*, 39, 4, 341–50.

Kahneman, D. and Frederickson, S. (2002) Representativeness revisited: attribute substitution in intuitive judgement, in T. Gilovich, D.W. Griffin, and D. Kaheman (eds) *Heuristics and Biases*, New York: Cambridge University Press.

Katz, I. (1991) Gordon Allport's 'The Nature of Prejudice', *Political Psychology*, 12, 1, 125–57.

Moon, J.D. (2006) Practical discourse and communicative ethics, in S.K. White (ed.) *The Cambridge Companion to Habermas*, Cambridge: Cambridge University Press.

Morgan, G. (2006) *Images of Organisation*, Thousand Oaks: SAGE.

Örtenblad, A. (2007) Senge's many faces: problem or opportunity? *The Learning Organization*, 14, 2, 108–22.

Powell, J.L. and Gilbert, T. (2008) Social theory and emotion: sociological excursions, *International Journal of Sociology and Social Policy*, 28, 9/10, 394–407.

Senge, P.M. (1990) *The Fifth Discipline, The Art and Practice of the Learning Organisation*, London: Random House.

Smith, P.A.C. and Sharma, M. (2002) Rationalizing the promotion of non-rational behaviors in organizations, *The Learning Organization*, 9, 5, 197–201.

Stacey, R. (2003) Learning as an activity of interdependent people, *The Learning Organization*, 10, 6, 325–31.

Stanovich, K.E. (1993) Dysrationalia: a new specific learning disability, *Journal of Learning Disabilities*, 26, 8, 501–15.

Stanovich, K.E. and West, R.F. (2000) Individual differences in reasoning: implications for the rationality debate? *The Behavioral and Brain Sciences*, 23, 5, 645–65; discussion 665–726. Online. Available www.ncbi.nlm.nih.gov/pubmed/11301544 (accessed 30 October, 2013).

Stanovich, K.E., West, R.F., and Toplak, M.E. (2011) Intelligence and rationality, in R. J. Sternberg and S. B. Kaufman (eds) *Cambridge Handbook of Intelligence*, New York: Cambridge University Press.

Venn, C. (1984) The subject of psychology, in J. Henriques, W. Hollway, C. Urwin, C. Venn, and V. Walkerdine (eds) *Changing the Subject*, London: Methuen.

Warnke, G. (2006) Communicative Rationality and cultural values, in S.K. White, (ed) *The Cambridge Companion to Habermas*, Cambridge: Cambridge University Press.

White, M. (2013) Higher education and problems of citizenship formation, *Journal of Philosophy of Education*, 47, 1, 112–27.

White, S.K. (2006) Reason, modernity and democracy, in S.K. White, (ed) *The Cambridge Companion to Habermas*, Cambridge: Cambridge University Press.

14 'Lexism' and the temporal problem of defining 'dyslexia'

Craig Collinson

This chapter examines the temporal problem of defining dyslexia. It is written by a 'dyslexic' seeking to challenge the dominant discourse of the non-dyslexic norm. That is to say, I question the existence of dyslexia, not the existence of dyslexics. The temporal problem of defining 'dyslexia' is part of a problem within our cultural perceptions of literacy. This includes the tendency to adopt the flawed conceptualisation of literacy as purely an ahistorical, technical, and educational tool separate from cultural context. In contrast, I adopt the 'ideological' model of literacy as a collective noun for a variety of cultural practices (Street, 1984). My argument is that our cultural preconceptions of literacy create a norm in relation to which dyslexics are judged abnormal.

The existence of a disability associated with being 'dyslexic' can be thought as distinct from the existence of the impairment 'dyslexia', which remains conceptually problematic. Individuals, who despite adequate education and intelligence struggle to acquire literacy skills, have long been recognised in the academic literature (Rice and Brooks, 2004), though 'dyslexia's' existence has proven conceptually problematic (Elliot and Gibbs, 2008). It is Lexism (i.e., normative practices, assumptions, and attitudes about literacy) that defines someone as a dyslexic and disables her or him, not a biological thing called 'dyslexia' (Collinson, 2012). Lexism, then, is a new concept that allows us to reconsider how dyslexics can be said to exist. I have previously posited an alternative model of dyslexia as a 'shadow concept' – whereby dyslexia can be thought of as a concept that is created, required, and disguised by another set of concepts surrounding literacy; that which I have termed Lexism (Collinson, 2012). In this chapter I examine historical aspects of 'Lexism', how its key features can be products of a given time and place.

In practice, dyslexics may need the term *dyslexia* to be recognised for acceptance and assistance (Riddick, 2001). However, when we recognise the existence of Lexism, the existence of dyslexics ceases to be reliant on problematic definitions of dyslexia. To investigate these conceptual issues, I examine and define the temporal problem of dyslexia in greater detail. I then outline historical evidence for early descriptions of literacy difficulties or dyslexic-like traits – one account from late seventeenth century England and two from antiquity, before the medicalisation of lower literacy levels from the late nineteenth century onwards

(Campbell, 2011). These accounts suggest that though social norms of literacy are not constant, the Othering of people deemed less literate but educated is part of our cultural inheritance. In order to illustrate my point I utilise the philosophical method of 'thought experiments' (Cohen, 2005; Baggini, 2005; Collinson, 2012).

The temporal problem

The temporal problem of dyslexia is that cultural norms and attitudes toward literacy change radically over time. *Temporal* in this instance should be taken to mean relating to time, and cultural norms of literacy are limited to a particular time period. The temporal problem of defining dyslexia has three main aspects: first, the difficulty of psychological assessments post mortem on individuals in the historical record; second, the shifting nature of norms of literacy by which dyslexics are judged abnormal, which means that dyslexics are not a biologically constant group; and third, the limited survival of relevant documentary evidence for earlier historical periods.

The first aspect of the temporal problem has been a matter of heated debate, especially over the identification of 'famous dyslexics' in the historical record (Thompson, 1971; Adelman and Adelman, 1987; Aaron et al., 1988; West, 1996; Thomas, 2000; Kihly et al., 2000). This academic debate has tended to assume a psycho-medical model of dyslexia built on the diagnosis of an individual post-mortem. It is certainly fair to argue that historical figures cannot be with any certainty assigned a 'dyslexic' identity as defined by psychologists. However, attempts to do so assume dyslexics are defined by 'dyslexia', for which there is neither clear definition nor conceptual clarity (Elliot and Gibbs, 2008). When dyslexics are defined as being Othered by Lexism, a new definition of dyslexics is possible – based on culture, not psychopathology (Collinson, 2012). Wider problems within disability historiography and the need to examine the role of Othering have been previously highlighted (Bredberg, 1999; Kudlick, 2003). It is for this reason that the popularity of 'famous dyslexics' on the internet could perhaps be seen as an 'invented tradition' or 're-use of the past' – part of the creation of self-identity recognised in historiography for other periods and for other social groups (Plumb, 1969; Finley, 1971; Finley, 1985; Hobsbawn and Ranger, 1992; Hen and Innes, 2000). This 'invented tradition' of famous historical figures might therefore be more usefully analysed as a construction of dyslexic identity, separate and distinct from psychological definitions.

The terminology used to describe people deemed less literate but educated changes over time, as do norms of literacy. However, the Othering is a common feature in societies with literacy based education and culture. For example, the very vague late nineteenth and early twentieth century term *feeble minded* was used to encompass what is now defined by a multitude of different 'impairments', including 'dyslexia' (Bennison, 1987; Franklin, 1994; Baker, 2002). But the earliest descriptions of dyslexia sought to separate the definition of people deemed intelligent but less literate from the definition of 'feebleminded' (Campbell, 2011). A lack of literacy was seen by European explorers and imperialists as a demarcation of the alien, the savage, the primitive, and the Other (Harbsmeier, 1989). Literacy in this period was, therefore, part of the justification for European superiority that underpinned wider racist ideologies and agendas, such as 'Social Darwinism', 'Eugenics', and the promotion of the medical concept of 'Feeble mindedness' (Thompson, 1998; Carey, 1992). It has been argued that dyslexics were seen in the later nineteenth and early twentieth century as the primitive/ savage/abnormal, as opposed to the non-dyslexic as the civilised/intelligent/ normal (McPhail and Freeman, 2005), and the role of mass literacy in the medicalisation of people deemed less literate in the later nineteenth century has been highlighted (Campbell, 2011). Such beliefs are expressions of literacy as purely a technical tool that associate literacy with rationality and 'full humanness' (Street, 1984).

The second aspect of the temporal problem of defining dyslexia is more significant. It has been argued that there are 'multiple literacies' (Street, 1984; Street, 1995), and we could add that there are multiple forms of any given type of literacy across different periods of its existence. English as a written language is not a historical constant and neither, therefore, would a dyslexic's difficulties with that language be unchanging (Riddick, 2001). Likewise, the dominant social form of literacy preferred by the elite is not constant; its normative practices and assumptions change with it. 'Dyslexics' can be defined as those judged 'abnormal' on a cultural level, but such norms are not a historical constant. As such, dyslexic identity can be thought of as similar to, but not the same as, definitions of ethnicity. In both cases the boundaries are drawn by social norms and attitudes within a culture, based on myths of difference, of 'us' and 'them', the norm and the Other.

The problem of applying biological norms to the social practice of literacy has been widely recognised in the field of dyslexia. It has been argued that there is no evolutionary norm of literacy and that dyslexics are defined by their failure to meet social expectations of literacy (Waber, 2001); that there is no evidence of literacy having any form of biological norm attached to it by which dyslexics can be defined 'abnormal' (Stanovich, 1994); that 'dyslexia' represents the lower end of 'normal' reading' (Shaywitz et al., 1992); and that reading is not a 'natural' process anyway (Reid-Lyon, 2001). The temporal problem of defining dyslexia is, therefore, part of a general problem in how we might define 'dyslexia'. It might also be a consequence of our cultural misconception of 'literacy' as a single monolithic thing, rather than perhaps a collective noun for 'multiple literacies' (Street, 1984; Street, 1995).

Social elite groups have continued to raise normative expectations of literacy and medicalise the failure to meet such norms (Carey, 1992; Payne, 2006; Campbell, 2011). In the late nineteenth and early twentieth century, great importance was attached to agendas linking the medical profession's development and government's desire for mass literacy (Campbell, 2011). Professional elites continued from the 1960s onwards to raise normative expectations of literacy (Payne, 2006), and there was growth in literacy in the United Kingdom after the 1870 Education Act created a fear among some British intellectuals that their social status was under threat (Carey, 1992). This in turn led to higher and higher levels of literacy being seen as necessary to convey erudition. This discourse, along with the expansion of education during the 1870s, led to artificial elevation of the social norm of literacy in Britain in the later part of the nineteenth century. Literacy as elite practice, therefore, raised the norms and expectations of literacy still higher. These discussions of literacy and literature were part of the wider eugenics debate (Carey, 1992). Indeed, the changing cultural concepts of literacy create and replicate norms of literacy that are not 'scientific' or 'biological' yet are often portrayed as such.

The limited sources in some periods of history, the third aspect of the temporal problem, mean that we cannot be sure of the percentage of the population that was literate or indeed what 'literate' meant in a given time or place. Nor can we be sure of the extent to which historical figures did or did not meet the norms and expectations of literacy in their own society or social group. The identification of such individuals in the historical record, therefore, is based not on a psychological assessment but *the perception* of a process of Othering. Likewise, the historical figures identified on the internet as 'dyslexic' are considered from the limits of historical evidence as not meeting the norms and expectations of literacy within their own cultural context. Nevertheless, this evidence is unlikely to satisfy a psychologist. The shifting norms of literacy over time would make attempts at psychological analysis of historical figures futile; while the Othering of people deemed less literate in different time periods is relatively constant, there is no constant of literacy to test against.

Early historical sources

It is important to highlight the role of norms of literacy in different periods and cultures in the Othering of people deemed less literate. Clear analysis of early scientific investigations of dyslexia has been provided elsewhere (Campbell, 2011), so rather than rehearse that argument here, I set out evidence of three sources that predate the discussion of the medicalisation of literacy. First, I consider an early scientific description of literacy difficulties found in the popular press, from late seventeenth century England. The second and third sources are from antiquity, early factual and fictional accounts of literacy difficulties that are suggestive of dyslexic-like traits. The purpose here is to highlight the role of our cultural preconceptions of literacy (i.e., Lexism), rather than the medical construct of 'dyslexia'. Again, these texts do not constitute historical evidence that would satisfy a psychologist. We can, however, discern Lexism in the historical record even if we cannot discern 'dyslexics'. Moreover, if we define dyslexics not by dyslexia but as those Othered by Lexism, then it can be argued that this is historical evidence of what we might term 'proto-dyslexics' (i.e., individuals in the historical record who were Othered by norms of literacy before the term *dyslexia* existed or was commonly applied).

The *Athenian Gazette* (1693) noted the 'strange account of a Boy in Durham'. A school master had written into the newspaper to outline the boy's case and ask for advice – rather like a modern 'agony aunt' column. The boy was fifteen, a gentleman's son, healthy, and 'yet he is no Fool, he sees and hears as well as any Body … and sometimes he will give an Answer that looks like something of Wit'. In other words, despite the more modest expectations of literacy in the late seventeenth century, the teacher was intelligent enough to realise the boy was not simply stupid.

The school teacher noted that the boy 'by all the means that have hitherto, or could be used, could never yet be made to know his Letters'. The boy seemed to have 'in one thing … to have a strong Memory, and in another none at all'. The teacher describes unusual traits, such as the inability to remember what the letters of the alphabet are called. The boy had clear traits of short-term memory and sequencing issues, in strong contrast to his long-term memory and intellect. The teacher's account acknowledges the boy's inability to write (presumably spell) much beyond his own name. However, the teacher went on: 'He cannot remember what such Letters are call'd, but as soon as he hears them named, he will presently tell you what they spell, which ordinarily with Children is the harder Task'. The teacher was faced with a student who did that which was deemed difficult well, yet struggled with that part of literacy deemed easy and it was for this reason that the boy was considered notable and was to remain in the historical record.

The response to the teacher was to admit that 'this is a very odd sort of a Relation and it's enough to puzzle our Philosophy to give a positive Answer'. However, the newspaper did suggest two possible answers, both of which *attempt scientific* explanations. One answer was that the 'Fibres that run from the Eye to the Brain must be defective', that these fibres had some form of pathology either in their situation, or were impaired or obstructed: 'disabled from leaving any Impression on that part of the Brain where the Faculty of Memory does officiate; but if so this must be general, and the boy can remember nothing that he receives by the Sense of Seeing'. The suggestion was that a 'multisensory' or alternative technique may be of use, as in the case of the Bishop of Sarim (i.e., Salisbury) who had recorded the example of someone who was blind being given alphabetic letters made of wood to learn to spell. The newspaper's other answer referred to 'the Fancy of the Mother in the Act of Conception, the imagining of some unaccountable Antipathy to letters, etc and if so, there's no Remedy but patience, for all Tryals will prove ineffective'. Though this description may not be of a 'dyslexic', it was a less literate member of society Othered by social norms of literacy. The boy from Durham may therefore be a 'proto-dyslexic' in that he was someone Othered by Lexism before the term *dyslexia* existed.

One of the earliest factual descriptions of literacy difficulties is from the *Lives of the Sophists* by Philostratus (Book 2.1. 558). Bradua is described as a 'fool' by his father Herodes Atticus (Philostratus, 1921: 165). The account of Bradau is from the time of the Roman Empire (second century CE), and provides a description of dyslexic-like traits:

> He [Herodes Atticius] was offended with his son [Bradua] Atticus. He had been misrepresented to him as foolish, bad at his letters, and dull of memory. At any rate when he [Bradua] could not master his alphabet, the idea occurred

to Herodes to bring up with him twenty-four [slave] boys of the same age named after the letters of the alphabet, so he would be obliged to learn his letters at the same time as the names of the boys.

(Philostratus, 1921: 165)

It is important to note that Philostratus records that Bradua has poor short-term memory ('dull of memory'), difficulties with sequencing ('could not master his alphabet'), and literacy difficulties ('bad at his letters'). Furthermore, Herodes Atticus, immediately after this paragraph, is quoted as referring to his son as a 'fool', yet here it is said that Bradua 'was misrepresented to his father as being foolish'. In other words, Bradua was unfairly said to be stupid. Nor is this the first time this source has been interpreted in this way, for it has been suggested that 'perhaps nothing more can be detected in this than a plutocrat's reaction to a mild case of dyslexia in his son' (Harris, 1989: 249), and other conclusions have also been drawn (Papalas, 1981).

An early fictitious account of people deemed less literate can be found in 'The Schoolmaster' (dated to the 280s or 270s BCE) by the Greek poet Herodas (also known as Herondas). This poem tells the story of a boy's failure to learn to read and write despite adequate education and literate parents (Herondas, 1921). The Greek text is difficult, and obviously fictitious, but Buck's translation is suggestive of how difficulties with literacy would have been explained in antiquity. The boy, 'Kottalos', according to his mother Metrotima (or rather the words Herodas places in her mouth), makes phonetic mistakes and demonstrates poor memory (Herondas, 1921). Herodas has the school master, Lampriskos, assure Kottalos' mother, Metrotima, that the boy will be repeatedly beaten until he can read. In the poem, Kottalos is not only likened to a Phrygian (i.e., a barbarian), but he is also fit only to lead donkeys and worse even than a slave. It has been suggested that 'elementary education is thus almost seen as a requirement of Greekness' and that the 'mother in her anger implies that the only kind of male who has any right to be as illiterate as this boy would be a Phrygian' (Harris, 1989: 140). Contrary to this tentative conclusion that literacy was usually considered a difficult skill to acquire, it seems more logical to suggest that the boy was not considered to be typical and was deemed to have failed the norms of literacy and expectations within his social group. Kottalas, after all, is referred to as being an 'idiot' (Herondas, 1921). His failure meant he was seen to be defined as the Other, placing him outside his social and ethnic group, a non-Greek and therefore similar to a 'barbarian', slave, and a 'donkey boy'.

These three examples provide evidence of long-standing cultural norms of literacy that Other and discriminate against a minority of people deemed educated but less literate. We might term them 'proto-dyslexics'. However, these proto-dyslexics existed in very different cultural, historical, social, and educational contexts.

Joanne, Peter, and the time machine

To demonstrate the temporal problem further, we can use a thought experiment that contrasts the norms of written language against the biology of 'dyslexics' by placing into a time machine two people defined as dyslexic by today's norms. The first dyslexic, let us call her Joanne, belongs to the 4 per cent of the most 'severely' dyslexic of today's population. The second dyslexic, let us call him Peter, belongs within the 6 per cent of the 'moderately' dyslexic of today's population. Joanne and Peter are then transported back in time to an earlier period, in this case seventeenth-century England, when people spelt as they spoke. Would they both still be dyslexic? Their biology would obviously remain the same, yet the norms of English literacy would be very different (Ellis, 1993; Upward and Davidson, 2011). The concept of 'dyslexia' would not exist, yet the Othering of people deemed less literate would, though perhaps in a different form.

We could argue that in seventeenth-century England Joanne may indeed find herself to be still dyslexic (or less literate) yet she might be 'less dyslexic' than she was when she left the twenty-first century moments before. This would depend on whether she belonged to the most severely dyslexic 1 per cent or was only just within the 4 per cent criteria. Though Joanne still fails to meet the social expected norms of literacy, she is closer to them than she was before she got into the time machine. The extent may well depend on her biological make-up. In this case, Joanne remains dyslexic and we could argue that norms of literacy only had a limited effect. However, without the label *dyslexic* Joanne is now in danger of being seen as 'stupid' or 'lazy', in effect she might face more stigmatising attitudes than she did in the twenty-first century. The key feature, however, is the cultural changes in written and spoken English and its associated norms that have occurred between the seventeenth and twenty-first centuries.

Yet now consider Peter, who after travelling back in time meets the social expected norms of literacy. Let us assume that in the twenty-first century, Peter is defined as 'moderately' dyslexic (i.e., relatively more literate than Joanne but still less literate than current modern norms of literacy). Now, Peter, having only moments before been dyslexic, steps into the seventeenth century, and ceases to be 'dyslexic' (less literate) as we would understand it. Peter might feel dyslexic as part of his self-identity, by the Othering and discrimination he experienced before he got into the time machine. However, by the standards of the seventeenth century, he would meet age related expectations of literacy. In this case, though Peter's biology, his 'deficit', remains a constant, it is not the deciding factor in his meeting social norms of literacy.

In this thought experiment, in the case of both Peter and Joanne, it is the relationship between their biology and the norms of literacy that effects whether (or to what extent) someone may face dyslexic-like difficulties. The thought experiment highlights the temporal problem of attempting to argue that there is a biological *thing* called dyslexia.

Conclusion

The temporal problem of 'dyslexia' on one level is conceptual or philosophical, on another level, cultural or historical. In seeking to understand 'dyslexia' in the sense of the social model of disability, we are seeking to understand a cultural prejudice toward people deemed less literate but intelligent and educated. Arguably there is no historical constant by which to judge the biological differences we all have in our aptitude (or otherwise) with the written word. Today we refer to such individuals (myself included) as 'dyslexic'. In different historical contexts, different terminology and ideological frameworks have been used to conceptualise such individuals, whom we might term proto-dyslexics.

The wide range of literacy practices and norms ('multiple-literacies') means that dyslexics are not a historical or genetically constant group. To argue that dyslexics are a constant group would presuppose literacy as purely a technical tool, ahistorical, requiring no understanding of cultural context, and without temporal change. It has been demonstrated that this is a highly questionable conceptualisation of literacy (Street, 1984). The definitional problem of dyslexia arises partly from our unwillingness to engage and challenge these cultural preconceptions of literacy. It is not dyslexia that defines *my* sense of cultural identity as a dyslexic. Rather it is my experiences of Othering within my own cultural environment, similar in some ways to those discussed in the historical texts within this chapter: to misquote President Clinton, 'It's the culture, stupid'.

References

Aaron, P.G., Phillips, S., and Larson, S. (1988) Specific reading disability in historically famous persons, *Journal of Learning Disabilities*, 21, 523–45.

Adelman, K. and Adelman, H.S. (1987) Rodin, Patton, Edison, Wilson, Einstein: were they really learning disabled? *Journal of Learning Disabilities*, 20, 270–79.

Athenian Gazette (1693) Saturday, August 26: Issue 14.

Baggini, J. (2005) *The Pig that Wants to be Eaten; and Ninety-nine Other Thought Experiments*, London: Granta.

Baker, B. (2002) The hunt for disability: the new eugenics and the normalization of school children, *Teachers College Record*, 104, 663–703.

Bennison, A.E. (1987) Before the learning disabled there were feeble-minded children, in B.M. Franklin (ed.) *Learning Disability: Dissenting Essays*, London: Falmer Press.

Bredberg, E. (1999) Writing Disability History: problems, perspectives and sources, *Disability and Society*, 14, 2, 189–201.

Campbell, T. (2011) From aphasia to dyslexia, a fragment of a genealogy: an analysis of the formation of a 'medical diagnosis', *Health Sociology Review*, 20, 4, 450–61.

Carey, J. (1992) *The Intellectuals and the Masses: Pride and Prejudice among the Literary Intelligentsia 1880–1939*, London: Faber and Faber.

Cohen, M. (2005) *Wittgenstein's Beetle and Other Classic Thought Experiments*, Oxford: Blackwell.

Collinson, C. (2012) Dyslexics in time machines and alternate realities: thought experiments on the existence of dyslexics, 'dyslexia' and 'Lexism', *British Journal of Special Education*, 39, 2, 63–70.

Elliot, J.G. and Gibbs, S. (2008) Does dyslexia exist? *Journal of Philosophy of Education*, 42, 3–4, 475–91.

Ellis, A.W. (1993) *Reading, Writing and Dyslexia: A Cognitive Analysis*, New York: Erlbaum.

Finley, M.I. (1971) *The Use and Abuse of History*, Harmondsworth: Penguin.

Finley, M.I. (1985) *Ancient History: Evidence and Models*, Harmondsworth: Penguin.

Franklin, B.M. (1994) *Backwardness to At Risk: Childhood Learning Difficulties and the Contradictions of School Reform*, New York: State University of New York Press.

Harbsmeier, M. (1989) Writing and the Other: travellers' literacy, or towards an archaeology of orality, in K. Schousboe and M.T. Larsen (eds) *Literacy and Society*, Copenhagen: Akademisk Forlag.

Harris, W.V. (1989) *Ancient Literacy*, Cambridge: Harvard University Press.

Hen, Y. and Innes, M. (2000) *The Uses of the Past in the Early Middle Ages*, Cambridge: Cambridge University Press.

Herondas. (1921) *The Mimes of Herondas Rendered in English*, New York: Buck M.S.

Hobsbawn, E. and Ranger, T. (1992) *The Invention of Tradition*, Harmondsworth: Penguin.

Kihly, P., Gregerson, K., and Sterum, N. (2000) Hans Christian Anderson's spelling and syntax: allegations of specific dyslexia are unfounded, *Journal of Learning Disabilities*, 33, 506–19.

Kudlick, C.J. (2003) Disability history: why we need another 'Other', *The American Historical Review*, 108, 3, 763–93.

McPhail, J.C. and Freeman, J.G. (2005) Beyond prejudice: thinking towards genuine inclusion, *Learning Disabilities Research and Practice*, 20, 254–67.

Papalas, A.J. (1981) Herodes Atticus: an essay on education in the Antonine age, *History of Education Quarterly*, 21, 2, 171–88.

Payne, G. (2006) Re-counting 'illiteracy': literacy skills in the sociology of social inequality, *British Journal of Sociology*, 57, 2, 219–40.

Philostratus. (1921) *Philostratus: Lives of the Sophists*, in Philostratus and Eunapius *Philostratus: Lives of the Sophists. Eunapius: Lives of the Philosophers*, London: Harvard University Press.

Plumb, J.H. (1969) *The Death of the Past*, Harmondsworth: Penguin.

Rice, M. with Brooks, G. (2004) *Developmental Dyslexia in Adults: A Research Review*, London: National Research and Development Centre for Adult Literacy and Numeracy. Online. Available www.nrdc.org.uk/ (accessed November 20, 2009).

Riddick, B. (2001) Dyslexia and inclusion: time for a social model of disability perspective? *International Studies in the Sociology of Education*, 11, 223–36.

Reid-Lyon, G. (2001) Why reading is not a natural process, *Orton Insight*, Autumn, 1–5.

Shaywitz, S.E., Escobar, M.D., Shaywitz, B.A., Fletcher, J.M., and Makuch, R. (1992) Evidence that dyslexia may represent the lower tail of the a normal distribution of reading ability, *The New England Journal of Medicine*, 326, 145–50.

Stanovich, K.E. (1994) Annotation; does dyslexia exist? *Journal of Child Psychology and Psychiatry*, 35, 4, 579–95.

Street, B.V. (1984) *Literacy in Theory and Practice*, Cambridge: Cambridge University Press.

Street, B.V. (1995) *Social Literacies, Critical Approaches to Literacy in Development, Ethnography and Education*, London: Longman.

Thomas, M. (2000) Albert Einstein and LD: an evaluation of the evidence, *Journal of Learning Disabilities*, 33, 149–57.

Thompson, L.J. (1971) Language disability in men of eminence, *Journal of Learning Disabilities*, 4, 34–45.

Thompson, M. (1998) *The Problem of Mental Deficiency: Eugenics, Democracy and social Policy in Britain c1870–1959*, Oxford: Clarendon Press.

Upward, C. and Davidson, G. (2011) *The History of English Spelling*, Chichester: Wiley-Blackwell.

Waber, D.P. (2001) Aberrations in timing in children with impaired reading: cause, effect or correlate? in M. Wolf (ed.) *Dyslexia, Fluency, and the Brain*, Timonium: York Press.

West, T.G. (1996) *In the Mind's Eye: Visual Thinkers, Gifted People with Dyslexia and Other Learning Difficulties, Computer Images and the Ironies of Creativity*, New York: Prometheus.

15 Behaviour, emotion, and social attitudes

The education of 'challenging' pupils

Marie Caslin

This chapter is premised by the belief that in the United Kingdom pupils deemed challenging are subject to a disablist education system that has been strategically determined by adults. This system works to remove the pupils from mainstream education through a process of segregation, where they are placed in so-called special schools, or through exclusion, where they are placed in an alternative provision (Booth, 1996; DfE, 2010). The literature on this topic makes plain that, for these young people, placement into educational settings is difficult (Ofsted, 1999). The pupils often face chaotic educational journeys during which they encounter and experience a wide range of educational provisions (Pirrie and Macleod, 2009; Gazeley, 2010; Pirrie et al., 2011). So although for many years the government has focused on raising standards in schools, it is my contention that what many young people experience is a utilitarian approach to education that is centred on the target setting agenda (Adams, 2008). I illustrate that, despite the rhetoric and moves to more inclusive practices, little room exists for those deemed challenging (Carrington, 1999). That is to say, the adoption of the utilitarian approach leads to 'undesirable' pupils being excluded for the greater good of the school. Indeed, in addition to employing formal mechanisms of exclusion, schools have found unofficial (often illegal) methods to remove this group of young people.

What does it mean to be deemed challenging?

The number of young people identified as having Behavioural, Emotional, and Social Difficulties (BESD) is continually growing (Cooper, 2006). What constitutes BESD, and how and where young people so labelled should be educated, is still a cause for intense debate among researchers (see Cole, 1998; Cole and Visser, 1999; Daniels and Cole, 2002). Since 1944 the terminology employed within government publications to describe young people with behavioural difficulties has included *maladjusted* and *Emotional and Behavioural Difficulties* (EBD), as well as BESD (Frederickson and Cline, 2009). Indeed, a conspectus of the current literature base highlights that BESD is an imprecise term that has evolved and altered overtime (Cole and Visser, 2005).

The use of labels to describe young people deemed to have BESD has been a focus of concern and interest for many educational researchers (Kelly and

Norwich, 2004; Thomas 2005; Tobbell and Lawthom, 2005). The subtext of the BESD label implies that behavioural difficulties 'lie in deficit and deviance in the child' (Thomas, 2005: 61). Consequently, having a label 'explains away' the problem, which can lead to teachers, parents, and others believing that there is nothing they can do or could have done to prevent the young person developing BESD; if the teacher feels it is out of her or his control, he or she will not change the pupil's educational environment (Lauchlan and Boyle, 2007). The disablist labelling that is employed to describe this group of young people is clearly significant, then, as in many ways it determines how they are perceived. This is why a change in attitudes is so important, for schools must move away from seeing the pupil as the problem.

Despite the negative impact of labelling young people with BESD (Thomas, 2005; Lauchlan and Boyle, 2007), there are perceived benefits. Both parents and teachers actively seek some form of diagnosis for 'problem' children: it provides parents with the extenuating circumstances that guarantee acceptance to the right educational provision and allows teachers to reconcile the increasing tensions between performance and inclusion (Adams, 2008). One of the major 'conditions' associated with BESD is Attention Deficient Hyperactivity Disorder (ADHD), manifestations of which are closely linked to forms of persistent disruptive behaviour (Watling, 2004). The literature on ADHD frequently acknowledges that one of the main benefits for parents who receive a formal diagnosis for their child is that they are less likely to feel blamed by the school for their child's actions and behaviours (Cooper, 2005). A parent whose child is deemed challenging often feels responsible. When this occurs the diagnosis can be seen as a 'label of forgiveness' (Lloyd and Norris, 1999). There are also potential benefits to receiving a label for the young people themselves. When a young person is identified as having BESD, for example, he or she becomes entitled to legal rights bestowed by legislation for pupils with so-called Special Educational Needs (SEN) (Visser and Stokes, 2003).

Notwithstanding the alleged benefits, concerns have been expressed regarding the labelling of young people. Among these concerns is the stigma that is attached to young people once they have been given this label (Galloway et al., 1994; Jones, 2003). This is especially true for pupils identified as having behavioural difficulties. These young people are stigmatised in a way that is not the case for those who have so-called learning difficulties (Clough et al., 2005). Blame is not bestowed upon those who have Down's syndrome or cerebral palsy, yet considerable assumptions are made about pupils identified with BESD (Clough et al., 2005). They are viewed as 'manipulative, capable of controlling their actions and unwilling to comply with the work orientation of the school' (Clough et al., 2005: 11). Significantly (given legitimate concerns about the medicalisation of disability), the terms that surround challenging behaviour are unclear, not least because BESD is not an officially recognised medical diagnosis. The ambiguous nature of the 'condition' may lead to it being perceived as having less status than other learning difficulties.

When young people are identified as having BESD they are taken down a path that separates them, they become trapped in a 'cocoon of professional help'

(Thomas, 2005: 67). There is the danger that having a label may lead to teachers having lowered expectations of the pupil's educational ability (Lauchlan and Boyle, 2007), that he or she is defined by and reduced to the perceived impairment (Garland-Thomson, 1997; Bolt, 2012). Thus, the labels can have a detrimental impact on young people in terms of how they are perceived and treated by adults. Within the process of a pupil receiving the BESD label, they are silenced by adults who consider them to be 'helpless' and in need of support (Thomas, 2005). Rarely are the perspectives of this Othered young person taken into account:

> The process of understanding children to be not only irrational but also emotionally disturbed effectively condemns them to voicelessness. Being seen as irrational (rather than simply stupid) is particularly damning, for it means that you are deemed unworthy even of consultation about what is in your best interests.
>
> (Thomas, 2005: 71)

Professionals construct perceptions of how young people labelled with BESD are to be understood. The young people become marginalised as they are deemed unfit to socialise with peers (Sutcliffe and Simons, 1993; Gillman et al., 2000; Tobbell and Lawthom, 2005). They are removed from mainstream educational settings due to the behaviour they display in the classroom. They are deemed not to fit with the educational agenda and, despite the rhetoric of inclusion, remain on the outskirts of mainstream education. Thus, the labels attached to young people determine their educational trajectory. That is to say, it is adults who are responsible for determining how these young people are understood; the support young people receive, to some extent, depends on the teacher and the ethos of the school they attend.

So labels are something of a double-edged sword: young people require the label in order to access specialist support, but once they have obtained the label they are perceived negatively by some adults. This can lead to young people being removed from mainstream education (Sutcliffe and Simons, 1993; Gillman et al., 2000; Tobbell and Lawthom, 2005). Some pupils obtain the label, yet remain unable to access additional educational support (Lauchlan and Boyle, 2007). Either way, acquiring the BESD label shapes how the young person is perceived and disabling attitudes are often held by educators (Miller et al., 2002; Riley, 2004). Due to the ambiguous nature of the BESD label, the pupil, without access to educational support, becomes the educational equivalent of a 'revolving door patient', for he or she experiences a wide range of educational provisions.

The labels employed are in a constant state of flux, largely due to the continually evolving political agenda. It is worth keeping recent history in mind, then, for in the late 1990s, New Labour inherited an education system that was based on a market forces agenda. The ideal of equal opportunity was consigned to mere rhetoric as New Labour policy sought the commodification of education. With a focus placed on performance and league tables, schools were encouraged to compete in order to recruit students. They concentrated on attracting the 'easiest' and 'cheapest' to teach (Ball, 2004: 6). Indeed, pre-1997 exclusionary practices remained largely untouched and unmodified (Ball, 1999). Within this framework, pupils who had received the BESD label continued to be removed from mainstream settings as they were deemed undesirable.

The greater good of the economy continued to be viewed as being more important than the needs of the individual. The effect was that the 'learner' effectively became a 'worker in waiting', acquiring the knowledge and skills necessary to successfully participate in the commercial world (Tomlinson, 2005). Those who did not fit in with this agenda, such as pupils who displayed challenging behaviour, were rejected or removed as they potentially offered the school no financial or exam performance gain (Adams, 2008). For schools, emphasis continued to be placed on the production of 'docile bodies' that conformed to expected disciplinary norms (Foucault, 1979). Under the provider-client split, schools and teachers were encouraged to view pupils as objects of the education system that led them to be valued according to their commercial worth (Gewirtz, 2002).

Within New Labour's social exclusion agenda (DfEE, 1997), emphasis continued to be placed upon the improvement of 'standards' and the accountability of the school. Pupils designated as having a behavioural problem were not considered a priority. The focus of help was placed upon failing schools rather than the individual needs of the pupil (Armstrong, 2005). Despite the policy seeking to develop more inclusive practices, those labelled as challenging continued to be removed. In addition, counter to the radical social model of disability, there remained a focus on deficiencies lying within the pupil. It was the pupil who continued to be identified as the 'problem'. By attributing blame to the pupil the school alleviates itself of any responsibility: it is the pupil who is failing, rather than the school system failing the pupil.

Removal of the so-called challenging pupil

A number of mechanisms have been employed to remove pupils who are seen to present a challenge. Schools adopt a variety of approaches to remove 'unwanted' pupils depending on the level of the behaviours displayed. One of the most common techniques utilised is exclusion from school. Exclusion can vary in degree from pupils who are excluded from just a lesson to those who are permanently removed from school (Daniels and Cole, 2010). However, as schools come under increasing pressure to reduce the number of permanent exclusions, they turn to alternative forms of removing 'problematic' young people.

The terms *unofficial* and *informal exclusion* have been coined to describe methods employed by schools to discourage pupils from attending without actually having to go through the procedures of fixed term or permanent exclusion (Stirling, 1992; Stirling, 1996). These unofficial exclusions are referred to by euphemisms such as *extended study leave* or *reduced timetable* (Evans, 2010). Despite this form of exclusion being illegal, previous research has found numerous examples of schools unofficially removing unwanted pupils (Stirling, 1992, 1996; Gordon, 2001; Gazeley, 2010). As these exclusions are illegal they cannot be appealed, there is no requirement to send work home and the absent pupils do not appear on official records (Evans, 2010). Families often do not challenge these exclusions because they may not understand how to question school authority (Evans, 2010). This leaves parents and their children in an extremely vulnerable situation where they are dependent on educational professionals. The imbalance of power leaves pupils and parents effectively silenced.

Despite the notion of inclusion being a feature of the education system for over 40 years, these young people remain on the periphery of mainstream schooling (Armstrong, 2005; Tomlinson, 2005; Adams, 2008). This is why social attitudes are a particular concern. Pupils labelled with BESD are less likely to be accepted due to the behaviours they display in the classroom (Tobbell and Lawthom, 2005). They are considered to *be* rather than to *have* a problem (Heary and Hennessey, 2005). They are removed due to educators adopting a utilitarian approach:

> There is a continued tension between the needs of the one and the needs of the many within debates on inclusion. The debate is probably nowhere more sharply focused than in the area of the inclusion of children with BESD.
>
> (Ellis et al., 2008: 130)

Educators are required to put the needs of the majority first, resulting in the Othered, challenging pupil being removed from the class, ignored by the teacher, and subsequently excluded from the school. Recent emphasis on measurement of performance as a central pre-occupation in schools (Gillborn and Youdell, 2000; Torrence, 2002; Cassen and Kingdon, 2007) has had a damaging impact on the educational journey of young people who have received the BESD label (Gillborn and Youdell, 2000; Torrence, 2002; Cassen and Kingdon, 2007).

Previous researchers who have attempted to track the educational journeys of young people labelled with BESD have encountered difficulties piecing together their often chaotic trajectories (Pirrie and Macleod, 2009; Gazeley, 2010; Pirrie et al., 2011). This is because individual young people experience severely disrupted educational pathways that include a wide range of educational provisions, often for only a relatively short period of time (Gazeley, 2010; Pirrie et al., 2011). These challenges are further exacerbated by the fact that many of the pupils have particularly complex and unstable patterns of school attendance (Gazeley, 2010). The disrupted educational pathways and poor attendance are likely to have a detrimental impact on a pupil's pre-existing learning and social difficulties (Pirrie et al., 2011).

Despite the rhetoric, then, inclusion was never truly embraced by the New Labour government. The continued emphasis placed on targets and academic results prohibited teachers from ever being able to cater for the challenging pupil (Hodkinson, 2012). Traditionally, young people who presented with challenging behaviour were placed in segregated educational institutions, which included asylums (Garner, 2009). It is my contention that, despite the inclusion agenda, little has changed as the pupils continue to be removed from mainstream settings. There has been an increase in the number of pupils placed in special schools and therefore segregated (Rustmeier and Vaughan, 2005). Moreover, the impact of removing pupils from mainstream education has led to a 'dump and hope' model being developed with young people being placed in a range of alternative provisions.

Make do and mend

According to the literature it is clear that the pupils are simply not wanted. However, it is important to pause here and consider the position of the teacher in this apparent ethical dilemma. Teaching pupils who display behaviours deemed challenging can be exceptionally demanding, both in terms of the professional skills required to deliver lessons and the emotional energy needed to deal with disruptive behaviour (Swinson and Knight, 2007). In one study, pupil behaviour was identified as one of the key factors in dissuading potential teachers from entering the profession and could cause existing ones to leave teaching (Barmby, 2006). Thus, the impact government legislation has on the individual teacher's ability to support this group of young people should be considered.

A recent document, produced on behalf of the government, reviewed behaviour standards and practices in schools in the United Kingdom (Steer, 2009). Within these standards the importance of ensuring that newly qualified teachers have the confidence and skills to deal with more challenging pupil behaviours is stressed. Many newly qualified teachers entering the profession believe they are ill-equipped to teach those labelled with BESD (Garner, 1996; Avramidis et al., 2000). Teacher training via the Post Graduate Certificate in Education (PGCE) pays scant attention to issues of emotional and psychological wellbeing, and many teachers graduate with a poor knowledge of how to tackle these issues – in particular, challenging behaviour (Margo et al., 2008). Teachers, then, are being placed in an impossible situation: they have not been adequately prepared to support this group of pupils, yet they are expected to cater for their educational needs. This has led to many educators developing the utilitarian approach to pupils deemed challenging by removing them from the mainstream setting. It has been argued that this is due to external pressures being placed on teachers such as academic targets.

For all that, the evidence indicates that there are teachers who show a strong child-centred approach to teaching pupils labelled with SEN, with a commitment to helping the pupil. It has been noted that 'what mattered more (than the nature of the provision) were the degrees of skill and commitment shown by staff in any site of provision' (Daniels et al., 2003: 134). In one study, several of the teachers who participated had a good understanding of home circumstances (Gross and McChrystal, 2001). They had clearly made determined efforts to involve the family and showed much flexibility in seeking to accommodate and include the child. The study demonstrates the importance of teachers being aware of the needs of individual pupils and the positive impact this can have on a young person's educational journey. However, for teachers to feel able to meet the learning needs of these pupils they have to feel competent and confident to recognise BESD. Worryingly, research suggests that teachers do not feel equipped to do so (Visser and Stokes, 2003; Male, 2003; Grieve, 2009; Goodman and Burton, 2010).

The literature base indicates that teachers do not have a shared understanding of what the term *BESD* means, which leads to the concept of inappropriate behaviour becoming socially constructed (Visser and Stokes, 2003; Male, 2003; Grieve, 2009). In the majority of cases it is teachers who are responsible for identifying whether or not a pupil has additional learning needs and should receive assessment for SEN. However, teachers have indicated a need for specialist training on labels associated with BESD and an understanding of each of these conditions (Goodman and Burton, 2010). These issues make it difficult for educational professionals to arrive at a consensus as to whether a pupil has BESD. Furthermore, these ambiguities also have an impact on a teacher's confidence to identify SEN.

Teachers, then, play a key role in identifying young people who they feel require assessment. However, their judgements are likely to be subjective, based on their attitudes, as well as perceptions of certain behaviours and thresholds of social tolerance (McKay and Neal, 2009). It is important, therefore, to take into account the impact of environmental factors and context in determining whether a young person presents with BESD. The notion of 'behaviour in context' has been highlighted elsewhere (Hargreaves et al., 1975). The argument is that whether a social action is considered problematic or non-problematic varies according to person, place, and time. The way teachers view young people is informed by their personal value positions (Hargreaves et al., 1975). There is also a reflection of wider policy perspectives and pressures (Adams, 2008). Because teachers are not provided with adequate training (Goodman and Burton, 2010), they are left to rely on their own previous experience in providing support to this group of young people (Gray and Panter, 2000).

Conclusion

The current education system in the United Kingdom is laden with contradictions between exclusion and inclusion that leave little room for those who present with challenging behaviour. This chapter highlights that the current system is not working from the perspective of the pupil or the teacher. Indeed, changes need to be made to ensure teachers are empowered to support all children in their classroom, including those who are seen to present a challenge. But my main concern is that instead pupils are removed through the processes of segregation and exclusion. The result is a chaotic educational journey where the pupil is likely to experience a wide range of educational provisions. The point to stress is that fundamental to this whole problem are attitudes that become manifest in disablist labels that are vague from scientific, sociological, and educational perspectives. Progress, therefore, begins with a change in attitudes.

References

Adams, P. (2008) Positioning behaviour: Attention Deficit/Hyperactivity Disorder (ADHD) in the post-welfare educational era, *International Journal of Inclusive Education*, 12, 2, 113–25.
Armstrong, D. (2005) Reinventing 'inclusion': New Labour and the cultural politics of special education, *Oxford Review of Education*, 31, 1, 135–51.

Avramidis, E., Bayliss, P., and Burden, R. (2000) Student teachers' attitudes towards the inclusion of children with special educational needs in the ordinary school, *Teaching and Teacher Education*, 16, 2, 277–93.

Ball, S.J. (1999) Labour, learning and the economy: a 'policy sociology' perspective, *Cambridge Journal of Education*, 29, 2, 195–206.

Ball, S. (2004) Education for sale! The commodification of everything? *Annual Education Lecture. Institute of Education*, University of London, London, June 2004. Online. Available http://mykcl.info/content/1/c6/05/16/42/lecture-ball.pdf (accessed 22 October 2010).

Barmby, P. (2006) Improving teacher recruitment and retention: the importance of workload and pupil behaviour, *Educational Research*, 48, 3, 247–65.

Bolt, D. (2012) Social encounters, cultural representation and critical avoidance, in N. Watson, A. Roulstone, and C. Thomas (eds) *Routledge Handbook of Disability Studies*, London: Routledge.

Booth, T. (1996) Stories of exclusion: natural and unnatural selection, in E. Blyth and J. Milner (eds) *Exclusion from School: Inter-professional Issues for Policy and Practice*, London: Routledge.

Carrington, S. (1999) Inclusion needs a different school culture, *International Journal of Inclusive Education*, 3, 3, 257–68.

Cassen, R. and Kingdon, J. (2007) *Tackling Low Educational Achievement* (Joseph Rowntree Foundation). Online. Available www.jrf.org.uk/bookshop/ebooks/2063-education-schools-achievement.pdf (accessed 10 May 2011).

Clough, P., Garner, P., Pardeck, J., and Yeun, F. (2005) Themes and dimensions of EBD: a conceptual overview, in P. Clough, P. Garner, J. Pardeck, and F. Yeun (eds) *Handbook of Emotional and Behavioural Difficulties*, London: Sage.

Cole, T. (1998) Understanding challenging behaviour: a pre-requisite to inclusion, in C. Tilstone, L. Florian, and R. Rose (eds) *Promoting Inclusive Education*, London: Routledge.

Cole, T. and Visser, J. (1999) The history of special provision for pupils with EBD in England: what has proved effective? *Behavioural Disorders*, 25, 111, 56–64.

Cole, T. and Visser, J. (2005) *Review of Literature on SEBD Definitions and 'Good Practice'*, University of Birmingham, accompanying the 'Managing Challenging Behaviour' report published by OfSTED (2005). Online. Available www.ofsted.gov.uk (accessed 24 February 2009).

Cooper, P. (2005) Biology and behaviour: the educational relevance of a biopsychosocial perspective, in P. Clough, P. Garner, J. Pardeck, and F. Yeun (eds) *Handbook of Emotional and Behavioural Difficulties*, London: Sage.

Cooper, P. (2006) Setting the scene, in M. Hunter-Carsch, Y. Tiknaz, P. Cooper, and R. Sage (eds) *The Handbook of Social, Emotional and Behavioural Difficulties*, London: Continuum.

Daniels, H. and Cole, T. (2002) The development of provision for young people with emotional and behavioural difficulties: an activity theory analysis, *Oxford Review of Education*, 28, 2 and 3, 312–29.

Daniels, H. and Cole, T. (2010) Exclusion from school: short-term setback or a long term of difficulties? *European Journal of Special Needs Education*, 25, 2, 115–30.

Daniels, H., Cole, T., Sellman, E., Sutton, J., and Visser, J. with Bedward, J. (2003) *Study of Young People Permanently Excluded from School*. Report no. 405 DfES, London.

Department for Education (1981) *The Education Act*, HMSO, London: DfE.

Department for Education (2010) *Permanent and Fixed Period Exclusions from Schools in England 2008/09* HMSO, London: DfE.

Department for Education and Employment (1997) *Excellence in Schools*, HMSO, London: DfEE.

Ellis, S., Tod, J., and Graham-Matheson, L. (2008) *Special Needs and Inclusion: Reflection and Renewal*, Birmingham: NASUWT.

Evans, J. (2010) *Not Present and Not Correct: Understanding and Preventing School Exclusions*. Barnardo's. Online. Available www.barnardos.org.uk/not_present_and_not_correct.pdf (accessed 16 June 2009).

Foucault, M. (1979) *Discipline and Punish: The Birth of the Prison*, Harmondsworth: Peregrine.

Frederickson, N. and Cline, T. (2009) *Special Educational Needs Inclusion and Diversity*, Buckingham: Open University Press.

Galloway, D., Armstrong, D., and Tomlinson, S. (1994) *The Assessment of Special Educational Needs: Whose Problems?* London: Longman.

Garland-Thomson, R. (1997) *Extraordinary Bodies: Figuring Physical Disability in American Culture and Literature*, New York: Columbia University Press.

Garner, P. (1996) Students' views on special educational needs courses in Initial Teacher Education, *British Journal of Special Education*, 23, 176–79.

Garner, P. (2009) *Special Educational Needs: The Key Concepts*, London: Routledge.

Gazeley, L. (2010) The role of school exclusion processes in the re-production of social and educational disadvantage, *British Journal of Educational Studies*, 58, 3, 293–309.

Gewirtz, S. (2002) *The Managerial School: Post-welfarism and Social Justice in School*, New York: Routledge.

Gillborn, D. and Youdell, D. (2000) *Rationing Education: Policy, Practice, Reform and Equity*, Buckingham: Open University Press.

Gillman, M., Heyman, B., and Swain, J. (2000) What's in a name? The implications of diagnosis for people with learning difficulties and their family carers, *Disability and Society*, 15, 3, 389–409.

Goodman, R.L. and Burton, D. (2010) The inclusion of students with BESD in mainstream schools: teachers' experiences of and recommendations for creating a successful inclusive environment, *Emotional and Behavioural Difficulties*, 15, 3, 223–37.

Gordon, A. (2001) School exclusions in England: children's voices and adult solutions? *Educational Studies*, 27, 1, 69–85.

Gray, P. and Panter, S. (2000) Exclusion or inclusion? A perspective on policy in England for pupils with emotional and behavioural difficulties, *Support for Learning*, 15, 1, 4–7.

Grieve, A. (2009) Teachers' beliefs about inappropriate behavior: challenging attitudes? *Journal of Special Educational Needs*, 9, 3, 173–79.

Gross, J. and McChrystal, M. (2001) The protection of a statement? Permanent exclusions and the SEN code of practice, *Educational Psychology in Practice: Theory, Research and Practice in Educational Psychology*, 17, 4, 347–59.

Hargreaves, D., Hester, S.K., and Mellor, F. (1975) *Deviance in Classrooms*, London: Routledge and Kegan Paul.

Heary, C. and Hennessy, E. (2005) *Developmental Changes in Children's Understanding of Psychological Problems: A Qualitative Study*, presented at the Annual Conference of the Psychological Society of Ireland, November 2005, Galway, Ireland.

Hodkinson, A. (2012) Illusionary inclusion – what went wrong with New Labour's landmark educational policy? *British Journal of Special Education*, 39, 1, 4–11.

Jones, R. (2003) The construction of emotional and behavioural difficulties, *Educational Psychology in Practice*, 19, 2, 147–57.

Kelly, N. and Norwich, B. (2004) Pupils' perceptions of self and of labels: moderate learning difficulties in mainstream and special schools, *British Journal of Educational Psychology Society*, 74, 411–35.

Lauchlan, F. and Boyle, C. (2007) Is the use of labels in special education helpful? *Support for Learning*, 22, 1, 36–42.

Lloyd, G. and Norris, C. (1999) Including ADHD? *Disability and Society*, 14, 4, 505–17.

Male, D. (2003) Challenging behaviour: the perceptions of teachers on children and young people with severe learning disabilities. *Journal of Special Educational Needs*, 3, 3, 162–171.

Margo, J., Benton, M., Withers, K., and Sodha, S., with Tough, S. (2008) *Those Who Can?* London: IPPR.

McKay, J. and Neal, J. (2009) Diagnosis and disengagement: exploring the disjuncture between SEN policy and practice, *Journal of Research in Special Educational Needs*, 9, 3, 164–72.

Miller, A., Ferguson, E., and Moore, E. (2002) Parents' and pupils' causal attributions for difficult classroom behavior, *British Journal of Educational Psychology*, 72, 27–40.

Office for Standards in Education (Ofsted) (1999) *Managing Pupil Behaviour Principles into Practice: Effective Education for Pupils with Emotional and Behavioural Difficulties*. A report from the Office of Her Majesty's Chief Inspector of Schools London: OFSTED. Online. Available www.ofsted.gov.uk (accessed 5 March 2009).

Pirrie, A. and Macleod, G. (2009) Locked out: researching destinations and outcomes for young people permanently excluded from special schools and pupil referral units, *Emotional and Behavioural Difficulties*, 14, 3, 185–94.

Pirrie, A., Macleod, G., Cullen, M., and McClusky, G. (2011) What happens to pupils permanently excluded from special schools and pupil referral units in England? *British Educational Research Journal*, 37, 3, 519–38.

Riley, K. (2004) Voices of disaffected pupils: implications for policy and practice, *British Journal of Educational Studies*, 52, 2, 166–79.

Rustmeier, S. and Vaughan, M. (2005) *Segregation Trends in LEAs in England 2002–2004*, Bristol: CSIE.

Steer, A. (2009) *Learning Behaviour: Lessons Learned: A Review of Behaviour Standards and Practices in our Schools*, DCSF publications. Online. Available www.publications. dcsf.gov.uk (accessed 5 March 2010).

Stirling, M. (1992) How many pupils are being excluded, *British Journal of Special Education*, 19, 4, 128–30.

Stirling, M. (1996) Government policy and disadvantaged children, in E. Blyth and J. Milner (eds) *Exclusion from Education*, London: Routledge.

Sutcliffe, J. and Simons, K. (1993) *Self Advocacy and People with Learning Difficulties*, Leicester: NIACE.

Swinson, J. and Knight, R. (2007) Teacher verbal feedback directed towards secondary pupils with challenging behaviour and its relationship to their behaviour, *Educational Psychology in Practice*, 23, 3, 241–55.

Thomas, G. (2005) What do we mean by 'EBD'? in P. Clough, P. Garner, J.T. Pardeck, and F. Yuen (eds) *Handbook of Emotional Behavioural Difficulties*, London: Sage.

Tobbell, J. and Lawthom, R. (2005) Dispensing with labels: enabling children and professionals to share a community of practice, *Educational and Child Psychology*, 22, 3, 89–97.

Tomlinson, S. (2005) *Education in a Post-welfare Society*, Buckingham: Open University Press.

Torrence, H. (2002) Assessment, accountability and standards: using assessment to control reform of schooling, in A. Halsey, H. Lauder, P. Brown, and A. Wells (eds) *Education, Culture, Economy and Society*, Oxford: Oxford University Press.

Visser, J. and Stokes, S. (2003) Is education ready for the inclusion of pupils with emotional and behavioural difficulties: a rights perspective? *Educational Review*, 55, 1, 65–75.

Watling, R. (2004) Helping them out, *Emotional and Behavioural Difficulties*, 9, 1, 8–27.

Epilogue
Attitudes and actions

David Bolt

This book is based on some of the seminars that I have organised as Director of the Centre for Culture and Disability Studies at Liverpool Hope University in the United Kingdom. The centre has established an international reputation for its innovative work in bringing together the humanities and the social sciences, especially the disciplines of disability studies, cultural studies, and education studies. The book exemplifies this work by bringing our multidisciplinary and interdisciplinary approach to the topic of changing social attitudes toward disability.

The project represents an international collaboration of eminent, established, and early-career scholars. That is to say, based in Belgium, France, the United Kingdom, and the United States, a few of us have had our doctorates for a decade or so, but the majority have completed within the last five years (or else hope to do so very soon); some of us hold professorial, senior, or junior academic posts, while others work independently; and our work spans the humanities and the social sciences. It is my hope that this diverse collaboration makes for a fresh approach to an age-old problem surrounding disability. The overarching argument, as stated at the start of the book, is that changes in social attitudes toward disability must not be underestimated, but documented and endorsed. Our multidisciplinary and interdisciplinary approach gives a rich expansion of this important contention.

In my introductory chapter I suggest that ableism and disablism may be thought of as two sides of the same ideological coin: the one renders people who are not disabled as supreme; the other refers to attitudes and actions against people who are disabled. The book as a whole considers the ideology of ableism in relation to history, culture, and education as, for instance, David Doat reveals an ableist anthropology that underlies much scientific work on evolutionary theories, Alex Tankard and Tom Coogan critique the ableist correction of cultural representation, and Alan Hodkinson illustrates a grand narrative of ableism in a virtual educational setting. Specific types of ableism are critiqued, too, as in Catherine Prendergast's chapter, which responds to sanism (see also Chapter 10 on ocularcentrism and Chapter 14 on lexism).

The concepts of ableism and disablism are interrelated, for ableism designates and defines the Other whom disableists avoid and attack. According to Craig Collinson, for example, dyslexics are Othered by lexism, a sociocultural process into which Sue Smith gains related insights by engaging with shifting representations of the cyborg soldier, and one that Owen Barden's chapter investigates on an institutional scale. Indeed, the book's multidisciplinary and interdisciplinary approach to attitudes reveals a truly diverse understanding of Otherness: Pauline Eyre shows how literature can represent the phenomenology of living as a disabled person without offering the reader a chance to render disability as Other, Claire Penketh critiques a number of academic papers that place their authors as observers of the Other (i.e., of the art students who have their work subjected to a form of diagnostic evaluation), Marie Caslin shows how the Othering of pupils deemed challenging moves effortlessly from labelling to exclusion, and I contend that people who have visual impairments are Othered by an ocularcentric social aesthetic.

In my introductory chapter I refer to the primary concern about researching disability, the danger of contributing to the ableist or even disablist social attitudes that we want not only to document but also to change. Emmeline Burdett illustrates this problem vividly in her critique of the responses of Anglo-American historians of Nazism to the Nazis' so-called euthanasia programme that tend to reflect stereotypical attitudes toward disability, something Alice Hall's chapter explores in relation to recent war photography. Indeed, the primary concern about researching disability is implicit if not explicit throughout the book.

In an endeavour to address this concern in our own work, we all adopt textual methodologies that are less likely to objectify people who are disabled, but this approach raises other concerns about understandings that may seem remote from experience. It is therefore worth emphasising that the value of disability memoir is recognised explicitly by Stella Bolaki (see also Chapter 5). In addition I should perhaps mention that we identify variously as having depression, dyslexia, multiple sclerosis, spina bifida, and visual impairment, among other things. That is to say, the majority of us have direct experience of social attitudes toward disability.

Given the nature of the field in which we work, moreover, our experiential knowledge is often supplemented by something less direct but still important. In order to illustrate this point I return once again to something mentioned in the introductory chapter. I have used guide dogs for decades and so am well aware that, in spite of legislation, people who are disabled can indeed be made unwelcome in restaurants that are owned or managed by people who have disabling attitudes. A consequence of my experience is that when I find somewhere less disabling, I become quite a loyal customer. Accordingly, at the end of a recent disability studies conference that I arranged with some of my colleagues, my partner and I dashed off to one of these favoured restaurants for a celebratory meal.

Within a few minutes of sitting down, I was contacted by one and then another colleague. They were thinking of joining us, so, given that we had not booked anything, I checked with the restaurateurs that space could be made for a few guests around our table. I mentioned that we would need a little extra room because some of us used wheelchairs and others used guide dogs. The restaurateurs did not hesitate to oblige, even though I was not sure exactly how many of the delegates would be joining us. Over the next half hour, two people became four, and then four became fourteen.

One of my colleagues was using a wheelchair and she arrived at the table without encountering any major problems. However, the same could not be said about another colleague who was using a power chair. The restaurant has an awkward porch that made it difficult for him to enter. Although my standard response to such situations is to leave and not return, in this instance, because our arrivals were staggered and some of us were already eating, I was more hesitant.

It was then that the importance of attitudes toward disability became apparent. The physical environment was practically deficient, ableist we might say, but the attitudes of the restaurateurs were far from disablist. More than being swiftly provided with a barely adequate ramp, my colleague was genuinely welcomed and joined the rest of us after a few minutes. I realise that such a positive attitude toward disability is not always sufficient, but in this instance it was a necessary condition of our enjoyment.

In contrast, around the same time my partner told me about something she witnessed on her bus journey home. The first point to stress is that the bus was accessible. This factor was particularly relevant because a man and a woman got on the bus and the latter was of short stature. However, the problem was that the bus driver automatically addressed the man and openly joked that he might only need to pay for one and a half adults, rather than two. Such disablist infantilisation is common yet profound. The eugenic implication is that a woman of short stature is childlike and thus an inappropriate love interest for any adult. In this example of anomalous practice, then, the so-called joke had disturbing connotations that clearly problematised the bus company's policy of accessibility.

These anecdotes are indicative of the major concern about social attitudes toward disability; they refer to social encounters that resonate with what are, in some senses, in some minds, far bigger issues. For example, while problematic Western ideas may be challenged by Hinduism, Buddhism, and Islam (Miles, 1992), faith communities surely need to change the ways in which disability is conceived and discussed if they are to welcome people who are disabled as full participants (Reynolds, 2012). A number of questions spring to mind, here. Why is a profound understanding of disability incompatible with the content of so many sermons? Why are so many religious metaphors fundamentally ableist if not disablist? Again, though admittedly not sufficient, changes in social attitudes toward disability prove a necessary condition of accessibility.

So in this book we take a critical approach to historical, cultural, and educational studies in order to document and demand changes in social attitudes toward disability. After all, ableist and disablist attitudes must be challenged and changed before actions can become truly meaningful. An accessible bus on the streets of twenty-first-century Britain is manifestly indicative of policy and legislation, not to mention actions, that depart from ableism. However, the situation remains problematic when a bus driver draws on disablist discourse to make a cheap joke. The thing is that, though perhaps no longer shut out physically, people who have impairments continue to be Othered through ableist and disablist attitudes in such everyday encounters.

References

Miles, M. (1992) Concepts of mental retardation in Pakistan: toward cross-cultural and historical perspectives, *Disability, Handicap and Society*, 7, 3, 235–55.

Reynolds, T.E. (2012) Theology and disability: changing the conversation, *Journal of Religion, Disability and Health*, 16, 1, 33–48.

Contributors

Owen Barden is Lecturer in Education at Liverpool Hope University, United Kingdom. He completed his EdD in 2011 at the University of Sheffield. He is currently working on several studies examining the relationships among dyslexia, digitally mediated social networks, and emerging literacy practices.

Stella Bolaki is Lecturer in the School of English at the University of Kent, United Kingdom. She completed her PhD in 2007 at the University of Edinburgh. She is author of *Unsettling the Bildungsroman: Reading Contemporary Ethnic American Women's Fiction* (2011) and is currently writing a book on illness narratives.

David Bolt is Senior Lecturer at Liverpool Hope University, United Kingdom. He completed his PhD in 2004 at the University of Staffordshire. He is author of *The Metanarrative of Blindness: A Re-reading of Twentieth-century Anglophone Writing* (2014) and editor, with Julia Rodas and Elizabeth Donaldson, of *The Madwoman and the Blindman: Jane Eyre, Discourse, Disability* (2012). He is also Director of the Centre for Culture and Disability Studies; Editor in Chief of the *Journal of Literary and Cultural Disability Studies*; Book Series Editor, with Elizabeth Donaldson and Julia Rodas, of Literary Disability Studies; and Founder of the International Network of Literary and Cultural Disability Scholars.

Emmeline Burdett is an independent scholar based in the United Kingdom. She completed her PhD in 2011 at University College London. She is currently working on Stefan Zweig's 1939 novel *Beware of Pity*.

Marie Caslin is Lecturer in Education at Liverpool Hope University, United Kingdom. She completed her PhD in 2012 at Liverpool John Moores University. She is currently working on an examination of the culture of blame that is a prominent feature of the educational journeys of pupils identified as having Behavioural, Emotional, and Social Difficulties.

Craig Collinson is Academic Support Officer at Edge Hill University, United Kingdom. He completed his MPhil in 2008 at the Graduate Centre for Medieval Studies, University of Reading. He is currently working on his doctorate at Edge Hill University.

Tom Coogan is Teaching Fellow in Management in the Business School at the University of Birmingham, United Kingdom. He completed his PhD in 2008 at the University of Leicester. He is guest editor, with Rebecca Mallet, of a special issue of the *Journal of Literary and Cultural Disability Studies* that focuses on comedy and disability (2013).

David Doat is Full Assistant at Lille Catholic University, France. He completed his MA in 2006 at the Catholic University of Louvain-la-Neuve. He is currently working on his doctorate at the University of Namur, Belgium.

Pauline Eyre is an independent scholar based in the United Kingdom. She completed her PhD in 2010 at the University of Manchester. She is currently working on literary representations of disability with a focus on disrupting Anglophone bias.

Alice Hall is Lecturer in Contemporary and Global Literature in the Department of English and Related Literature at the University of York, United Kingdom. She completed her PhD in 2010 at the University of Cambridge. She is author of *Disability and Modern Fiction: Faulkner, Morrison, Coetzee and the Nobel Prize for Literature* (2012).

Alan Hodkinson is Associate Professor at Liverpool Hope University, United Kingdom. He completed his PhD in 2003 at the University of Lancaster. He is author, with Philip Vickerman, of *Key Issues in Special Educational Needs and Inclusion* (2009).

Claire Penketh is Senior Lecturer at Liverpool Hope University, United Kingdom. She completed her PhD in 2010 at Goldsmiths College, University of London. She is author of *A Clumsy Encounter: Dyspraxia and Drawing* (2011).

Catherine Prendergast is Professor at the University of Illinois at Urbana-Champaign, United States. She completed her PhD in 1997 at the University of Wisconsin at Madison. She is author of *Literacy of Racial Justice: The Politics of Learning after Brown v. Board of Education* (2003) and *Buying into English: Language and Investment in the New Capitalist World* (2008). She is guest editor, with Elizabeth Donaldson, of a special issue of the *Journal of Literary and Cultural Disability Studies* that focuses on representing emotion and disability (2011).

Sue Smith is University Tutor at the University of Leicester, United Kingdom, where she completed her PhD in 2010. She is currently working on the representation of disability and the cyborg soldier in 1980s American Culture.

Alex Tankard is Visiting Lecturer at the University of Chester, United Kingdom. She completed her PhD in 2010 at the University of Liverpool. She is currently working on disability and male-male intimacy in representations of Doc Holliday since c.1880.

Index

ableism, 3, 4, 5, 6–7, 15, 16, 22, 26, 62, 110, 113, 115, 121, 126, 127, 128, 172–23, 174
advertising, 4, 8, 52, 109, 110, 113–15
aesthetics, 8, 34, 54–55, 57, 92–94, 105, 109–10, 111–12, 113–16, 126, 136, 137, 173
agency, 6, 7, 30, 35, 60–61, 66, 93, 105
alterity, 110
amputees, 51, 56, 81, 83
anomalous practice, 1, 5, 6, 174
antibiotics, 27, 63, 65
antipsychiatry, 96
art, 8, 30, 43, 50, 54–55, 57, 73, 74–75, 95, 102, 112, 132–40, 173
asylum, 19, 38, 42–43, 166
avoidance, 8, 99, 139, 147

Barnes, Colin, 2, 4, 6, 110, 125, 143, 149
beauty, 30, 34, 54–55, 109, 110, 112, 114, 115
biomedicine, 28
body trauma, 80, 83, 84, 87
Bolt, David, i, 1, 3, 4, 18, 20, 99, 109, 132, 139, 145, 147, 164, 172, 176

castration, 112
Clough, Peter, viii, 128, 163
community, 2, 5, 8, 15, 16–17, 20, 21, 22, 95, 96, 101, 105, 112, 121–22, 150, 174
consumption, 27, 28, 30. *See also* tuberculosis
Couser, G. Thomas, ix, 89, 91
cure, 65, 78
cyborg, 80–82, 83, 84–87, 173, 177

Darwinism, 7, 15, 16–18, 19, 21, 22, 46, 155
Davis, Lennard, viii, 3, 101, 142

dependency: dependence, 16, 18, 20; independence, 20; interdependence, 7, 16, 17–19, 20
depression, 32, 64, 173
Disability and Society, 3, 4
disablism, 3, 4–7, 22, 125, 162, 163, 168, 172–73, 174
disease, 22, 26, 27, 29, 32–33, 38, 41, 65, 66, 77, 95
dismodernism, 101
Donaldson, Elizabeth, ix, 66, 176, 177
Down's syndrome, 8, 163
drugs, 7, 60, 61–65, 66, 94
dyslexia, 8, 22, 134, 136, 142, 153–55, 56, 157–60, 172, 173, 176

embodiment, 109, 113, 115–16
eugenics, 15, 16–17, 19–20, 21, 38, 41, 46, 155, 156, 174
euthanasia, 38–48, 101, 173

fear, 16, 26, 43, 45, 56, 62, 64, 76, 81, 86, 104, 125, 137, 145, 146, 149, 155
femininity, 84. *See also* gender
Finkelstein, Vic, 1–2, 18, 19–20
Foucault, Michel, 97, 134–35, 136, 165

Galton, Francis, 17, 28, 41
Garland-Thomson, Rosemarie, ix, 52, 53, 76, 114, 135, 147, 164
gender, 7, 80–84, 86–87, 139. *See also* femininity and masculinity
Goffman, Erving, 147
Goodley, Dan, viii, 22, 121, 143–44, 150

Habermas, Jürgen, 150–51
Hall, Stuart, 104
Hevey, David, 52–53, 54, 55
HIV/AIDS, 33, 63

Hodkinson, Alan, viii, 8, 121, 166, 172, 177
Hughes, Bill, 28, 56, 146
Hunt, Paul, 4
hygiene, 34, 45

identity, 26, 27, 28, 29, 35, 62–63, 72–73, 76, 77, 80, 81–85, 86, 94–95, 121, 127, 133, 135, 139, 140, 154–55, 159, 160
infantilisation, 174
institutionalism, 3, 39, 78, 96
International Journal of Art and Design Education, 132

Journal of Literary and Cultural Disability Studies, viii, 176, 177

Kudlick, Catherine, 39, 45, 47, 154
Kuppers, Petra, viii, 122

language: labeling, 1, 8, 22, 95, 113, 122, 159, 162–65, 166, 167–68, 173; metaphor, 53, 63, 65, 89, 99, 100, 104, 106, 125, 148, 174; person-first, 4; terminology, 3–4, 72, 154, 160, 162
learning difficulty, 3, 4–5, 6, 136–37, 142, 148, 163, 166. *See also* learning disability
learning disability, 4, 8, 78, 142, 147. *See also* learning difficulty
legislation, i, 1, 5–6, 163, 167, 173, 174
Lewiecki-Wilson, Cynthia, ix, 60
Linton, Simi, 62–63, 65
Longmore, Paul, 52, 54, 71, 73, 77
love, 17, 22, 84–85, 86, 112, 113, 174

masculinity, 81, 82–85. *See also* gender
medication, 61, 62–67, 92, 94, 97
medical model of disability, 26, 28, 29, 32, 33, 34, 35, 62, 63, 66, 90, 154
memoir, 7–8, 60–65, 89–92, 94, 97, 173
mental health problems, 5, 8, 94
Mercer, Geof, 4, 6, 125, 143
Merleau-Ponty, Maurice, 104, 106
Mitchell, David, viii, 2, 53, 75, 99, 114
Morris, Jenny, 39

narrative, 8, 15, 28, 53–54, 56, 62–63, 66, 75–76, 81–82, 83–84, 86–87, 89–94, 97, 99, 102, 106, 113, 114, 122, 124, 125, 126, 127, 128, 137, 147, 172, 176
Nazism, 7, 38–48, 173
neuropathology, 89

Norden, Martin, 85
normalism, 83, 94, 101–2, 105, 107, 126, 135–36, 137, 138
normate, 135

ocularcentrism, 109–10, 111, 112, 113, 114, 115–16, 136, 172–73
Oliver, Mike, 2, 4
organisations, 6, 57, 63, 94–95, 121, 122–23, 128, 134, 142, 143–45, 147–51
Otherness, 41, 45, 52–53, 81, 85–86, 100, 102, 110, 111, 113, 115, 121, 122, 127, 135–36, 138, 154–55, 156, 157, 158–59, 160, 164, 166, 172–73, 174

paleopathology, 21, 22
pathology, 21, 26, 28, 29, 30, 78, 89, 95, 132–33, 135, 136–37, 138, 157
Paralympics, 56
pariahs, 85
Penketh, Claire, viii, 8, 132, 133, 135, 173, 177
physiognomy, 28–29
physique, 26, 33
pity, 4, 26, 30, 35, 52, 62, 100, 113, 146, 176
policy, i, 1–2, 5–6, 48, 63, 66, 164, 165, 168, 174
postpsychiatry, 96–97
power: disempowerment, 73, 100; empowerment, 5, 99, 100, 104, 105, 107, 128–29, 139, 168
Prendergast, Catherine, 7, 60, 66, 89, 97, 172, 177
propaganda, 38, 41–42, 44, 71, 83
prosthetics, 53, 54, 56, 80–81, 83, 85, 86, 103, 125
psychology, 2, 76, 83, 84, 100, 103, 115, 142, 143–44, 145–46, 147, 149–50, 154, 156, 167
psychopathology, 96, 154

Quayson, Ato, viii, 105, 124, 126

rationality, 2, 8, 16, 19, 95, 127, 142–44
rehabilitation, 53–54, 56, 81, 83–84, 85, 87
Rodas, Julia Miele, ix, 4, 158, 176
romanticism, 35

schizophrenia, 8, 46, 60, 61–62, 65, 67, 89–90, 91–93, 94–96, 97
sentimentality, 26, 28, 30, 35, 53, 89
Serlin, David, viii, 80–81, 83

sexuality, 67, 84, 85
Shakespeare, Tom, 1, 4, 20, 21–22
Siebers, Tobin, ix, 50, 54–55, 57
Snyder, Sharon, viii, 2, 53, 75, 99, 114
social model of disability, 2, 4, 159, 165
Sontag, Susan, 53, 57, 63, 65
Special Educational Needs, 8, 132–33, 138, 139, 163, 167–68, 177
stereotyping, i, 6, 20, 28, 52–54, 110, 115, 121, 145, 146, 149, 150, 173
sterilisation, 38, 41
stigma, 3, 32, 35, 45, 57, 66, 85, 89, 91, 96, 103, 104, 110, 114, 135, 147, 159, 163
suicide, 32, 34

technology, 15, 18, 50, 56, 57, 80, 81–82, 83, 84, 86, 87, 96, 128, 137, 138–39
tuberculosis, 7, 26–27, 28, 32, 33–35. *See also* consumption

violence, 26, 30, 50–51, 52, 85, 86, 96
vulnerability, 6, 7, 15–16, 17–20, 29, 33, 47, 51, 52, 57, 86, 89, 103, 128, 166

Waldschmidt, Anne, viii, 101, 105
war, 6, 18, 38–39, 41, 42, 44, 51–53, 54, 55–56, 80–82, 83–87, 90, 91, 101, 103, 112, 173
weakness, 17, 20, 28, 32